D0474234

"Since the school closed in 1976, the idea of reopening it keeps coming up — with much interest especially from nursing. In 2002 Marilyn Chow, then VP for nursing at the national program, had Dr. Catherine Gilles from Yale do an analysis of the feasibility of reopening a school of nursing — perhaps in a partnership with a university. This was at a time of insufficient nursing programs in California, and would have contributed to easing the nursing shortage of the early 2000s. But it wasn't meant to happen then. More recently, with the new Kaiser Permanente School of Medicine expected to open in Pasadena in 2020, the idea of reinstating the school as part of the school of medicine keeps coming up as a topic — this time at the graduate level and contributing to the school of medicine's interdisciplinary education track. Will this come to fruition? Whether it does or not, the concepts and ideals of KFSN are now embedded within Kaiser Permanente and will be a part of the Kaiser Permanente School of Medicine."

—Claire O'Sullivan Lisker, R.N.*

*Personal communication of Clair O'Sullivan Lisker with Steve Gilford, December 2019, Berkeley, California.
Transcript on file at the Kaiser Permanente Archives, Oakland, California.

EDITORS

Deloras Jones

Jim D'Alfonso

LEAD AUTHOR

Steve Gilford

CONTRIBUTING AUTHORS

Deloras Jones

Jim D'Alfonso

Priscilla S. Javed

KAISER PERMANENTE'S ARCHIVIST

Lincoln Cushing

2020 ALUMNI ASSOCIATION EDITORIAL BOARD

Clair O'Sullivan Lisker, Class '51A

Janice Price Klein, Class '63

Sylvia Barnes Bertram, Class '64

Kathleen Walsh, Class '72

PRODUCTION TEAM

Terri Moss, Moss Communications

Nicole Watson, Pensé Design

Colleen O'Neill

Printing: Lynx Group

KAISER FOUNDATION SCHOOL *of* NURSING

A LEGACY OF DISRUPTIVE INNOVATION

1947-1976

EDITORS *Deloras Jones* | *Jim D'Alfonso*

Kaiser Foundation School of Nursing: A Legacy of Disruptive Innovation
©2020 by Moss Communications. All rights reserved. No part of this
book may be reproduced in any form or by electronic or mechanical means,
including information storage and retrieval systems, without the permission
from the publisher, except by a reviewer who may quote brief passages
in a review.

Library of Congress Cataloguing-in-Publication Data
Library of Congress Control Number: 2020908270

Jones, Deloras
D'Alfonso, Jim

Kaiser Foundation School of Nursing: A Legacy of Disruptive Innovation :
A history of the school of nursing and impact of its legacies for the nursing
profession and nursing education at Kaiser Permanente and globally.

Includes bibliographical references.
p.cm.

ISBN 9978-0-9833014-5-5

Printed in the United States of America
First Printing: 2020

Cover and interior design by Nicole Watson, Pensé Design

For permission and special ordering information, contact Jim D'Alfonso:

1714 Franklin Street, Suite 100-370
Oakland, CA 94612
jim.dalfonso@gmail.com
602.717.5400

To order books, please visit www.mosscommunications.net

ACKNOWLEDGEMENTS

This book was a labor of love; love that emerged from an inspirational vision and leadership that responded to the demands of the times in a way that disrupted the status quo and influenced the course of nursing education, the nursing profession and health care delivery. This book and the Kaiser Foundation School of Nursing (KFSN) were built on the shoulders of the faculty; the disruptive innovators who created an exceptional school of nursing, developed a cohort of 1,065 registered nurses over 30 years and shaped its legacy elements influencing Kaiser Permanente (KP) nursing to this day.

We wish to acknowledge the KFSN Editorial Board, the Legacy Committee, and the KFSN Alumni Association Board of Directors, who brought to life the history of KFSN. The Board served as the voice of the alumni and provided continuous encouragement and support for this important endeavor; they provided the vision of "Continuing the Legacy." In addition to Janice Klein and Jackie Anderson, the Board also served as the Legacy Committee.

We are deeply indebted to the Kaiser Permanente executive leadership, and in particular, Bernard Tyson, president and CEO of Kaiser Permanente at the time of his passing, for his heartfelt commitment and support of the memory of KFSN and the alumni association. Tyson launched the KFSN book project with a substantial grant allowing us to create a sculpture that now stands at the entrance of KP Oakland Medical Center, and in turn led to the genesis of the book.

The stories and voice of KFSN alumni came to life when Steve Gilford, as respected Kaiser historian, eagerly embraced the challenge to close a known gap in the telling of the history of Kaiser Permanente by revealing this story of KFSN. We thank the alumni and Kaiser Permanente leaders whose oral histories and responses to the questionnaires allowed Gilford to gather historical information and then narrate the story and legacy elements. Our gratitude extends to Clair Lisker for her unfailing ability to fill in the historical milestones and help weave together the narrative. We are grateful to Kaiser's early physicians and administrators, who envisioned and valued the kind of nurses graduates became, knowing we were prepared to practice nursing in a manner that actualized the Permanente Way and its disruptive vision of total health, while setting the standard for future Kaiser Permanente nurses to follow.

We are indebted to our content developers and editors who emerged as a committed team to produce this important historical narrative, including Terri Moss, Nicole Watson, Colleen O'Neill and Lynx Group.

The guiding lights and driving forces behind this book were Jim D'Alfonso and Deloras Plake Jones. Together, they made a dynamic and unstoppable duo. As champion and visionary, Dr. D'Alfonso led the effort, deeply understanding that KFSN was undeniably the ancestral origins of Kaiser Permanente's present-day innovative and disruptive nursing workforce, and the essential framework for academic advancement, professional development, clinical excellence and health systems transformation now reimagined and thriving across the enterprise and within the KP Scholars Academy.

Jones' tireless leadership and energy was a *tour de force*. Her passion and commitment to nursing willed this loving tribute into being. Through her resolve and drive, Jones knew that by describing the foundations upon which Kaiser Permanente's present-day nursing culture and vision were built, this story could rekindle a passion in nursing and inspire future nurse leaders within KP and beyond. We trust the reader will find she was absolutely right!

— The Kaiser Foundation School of Nursing Alumni Association

CONTENTS

Dedication

This book is dedicated to the enduring legacy of Kaiser Foundation School of Nursing faculty and alumni and all nurses, nurse educators and Kaiser nurses who share their passion for professional nursing and follow in their footsteps.

Proceeds from the sale of this book benefit the KFSN Alumni Association's Scholarship Fund.

SUSAN V. BOSAK

"Legacy is about learning from the past, living in the present and building for the future. It is constructed over time and is what one is remembered for when one is gone."

PROLOGUE

The story of the Kaiser Foundation School of Nursing (KFSN) is a reflection of pioneers and legends that made a difference and had an enduring impact on the profession while transforming clinical practice and systems in Kaiser Permanente (KP) for more than 70 years. KFSN nurses were leaders of disruptive innovation, and they helped realize a new way of viewing health care through the lens of Kaiser Permanente's provocative medical model, which focused on wellness rather than illness.

Kaiser nurses were considered essential to the success of implementing the KP vision and mission for total health. In realizing this role and boldly transforming practice settings, they influenced the world of integrated nursing and holistic practices for patients, families and communities across the continuum of care. Their contributions did not just build upon previous successes; rather, the innovations they championed ushered in a new era of professional nursing that continues to thrive today. KFSN nurses and Kaiser nurses launched bold transformation while building a legacy of academic excellence, diversity, resilience and a professional practice model that has endured the test of time.

As the World Health Organization celebrates 2020 as the "Year of the Nurse and the Midwife," it is an opportunity for all nurses to reflect on their journey and contributions to the wellness of a global community. The legacy of KFSN, and the pioneers that led by entering nursing through its doors, is a reflective journey of deep purpose and promise. A small yet incredibly powerful group of nurses, driven by professional ethics and caring science values, delivered on the promise of total health — and in doing so blazed a trail for all nurses who followed them into the profession.

Former Kaiser Permanente Medical Director for Total Health Dr. Ted Eytan shared his belief in 2017 about the power of KFSN and its graduates in this way: "Kaiser nurses were practicing the kind of medicine in the 1950s that we are trying to get to today."[1]

The proud legacy of KFSN graduates lies in their continued presence, relevance and influence in Kaiser Permanente today. A statue of a KFSN student holding an infant was erected and dedicated during the opening of the new Kaiser Oakland Medical Center in 2015 (the original home of KFSN), and visitors can peruse a display case of KFSN memorabilia and period pieces located near the lobby entrance, commemorating the profound impact of KFSN nurses in the pursuit of world-class care through their steadfast dedication to excellence.

Over the years, KFSN graduates clearly have articulated and embodied the voice of visionary nurses advancing beyond the social and professional practice norms of their time. Alumni have distinguished themselves as pioneers and disruptive innovators in nursing education and clinical practice. KFSN and the many contributions of its nurses defined who we are as Kaiser nurses, and their legacy informs us and serves as a model for success in advancing new concepts in professional nursing practice, education and systems transformation within the nation's largest not-for-profit integrated health care system.[2]

The genesis of this book is the direct result of a desire to capture stories and share the voices of KFSN's legacy as a cherished source of context, relevance, pride and inspiration for all Kaiser nurses. Since 2013, the partnership between KFSN alumni, Kaiser Permanente (KP) executive leadership and the newly created KP Scholars Academy has resulted in an award-winning documentary on KFSN, presentations at national and international nursing conferences, a peer-reviewed publication and, most importantly, a renewed interest in the deeper value of KFSN's disruptive legacy in honoring our past, inspiring our present and co-creating the future of Kaiser nursing for generations to come.

The genesis of this book is the direct result of a desire to capture stories and share the voices of KFSN's legacy as a cherished source of context, relevance, pride and inspiration for all Kaiser nurses.

Our hope for this book is that through the inspirational stories of KFSN graduates and faculty, captured through interviews and archival research, all nurses experience a deep pride in their profession. We seek to lead Kaiser nurses in particular to find a revitalized sense of shared purpose, connection to the history of Kaiser nursing and a renewed commitment to the journey of total health.

Kaiser nurses have a rich history of ensuring access to affordable and timely care. They breathe life into the Kaiser Permanente mission and vision every day as they endeavor to advance high-quality care in the diverse communities we serve.

Our history reflects a passion for professional nursing that makes a difference. This passion — our ability to see unique opportunities when faced with obstacles and our commitment to act in new and radical ways — is in our collective DNA. That devotion to excellence over time demonstrates that the disruptive innovations we pioneer today can inform and transform care and healing environments for generations to come.

Deloras Jones, MSN, RN
Class of 1963 and Retired Health System Chief Nurse
Executive, Kaiser Permanente, Oakland, California

Jim D'Alfonso, DNP, RN, Ph.D.(h), NEA-BC, FNAP
Executive Director, Professional Excellence
The KP Scholars Academy,
Kaiser Foundation Hospitals and Health Plan,
Oakland, California

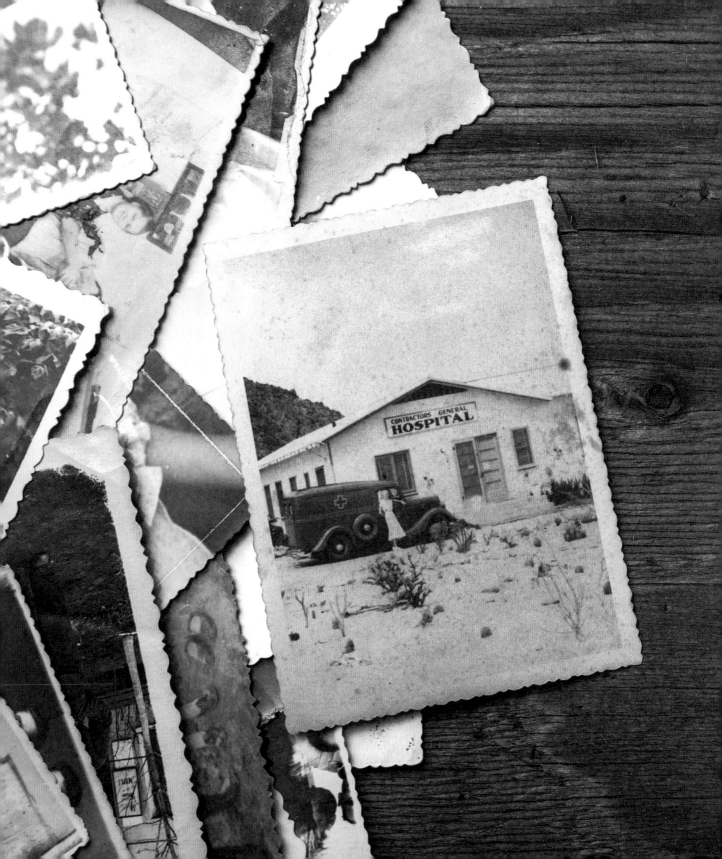

BEFORE the BEGINNING

NECESSITY IS THE (1) MOTHER OF INVENTION

The Foundation of Kaiser Health Care's
Culture of Disruptive Innovation

FALL 1933 – FOURTH YEAR OF THE GREAT DEPRESSION Betty Runyen, RN, was excited and a bit nervous.[1] Her brother had offered to drive his 21-year-old sister to her new job at a small wood frame hospital, Contractors General, at a work camp in the midst of the California desert about 130 miles east of Los Angeles.

Adventurous by nature, Runyen had liked the idea of working in this remote 12-bed hospital, taking care of 5,000 construction workers who were digging and tunneling a 242-mile aqueduct to bring Colorado River water to a rapidly growing Los Angeles. She was sure this would be more exciting than working with new mothers in Labor and Delivery at the 225-bed Methodist Hospital in Los Angeles, where she had trained as a diploma nurse.

They turned off the paved highway and bounced up a dirt road that ran across a dry stream bed. Ten bumpy minutes later they arrived at their destination, the Dixon-Bent work camp, and the little hospital where she was greeted by Dr. Sidney Garfield.

Garfield had hired her sight unseen, though his partner, Dr. Eugene Morris, had worked with her on an ad hoc basis. The 27-year-old surgeon from Los Angeles County General Hospital only recently had opened this tiny, temporary hospital; her arrival meant now he had a nurse. Until then, the entire hospital staff had consisted of Garfield and Cal and Helen Corbett, the husband-and-wife team that served as orderly/ambulance driver and cook/housekeeper.

Obviously proud of his modest facility, Garfield showed Runyen around. She saw it was well-equipped, and that Garfield took painstaking measures to make patients as comfortable as possible. Rather than the typical sterile white decor, the hospital was painted in warm pastels and was air-conditioned, a rarity in 1933. Garfield later would recall, "We try to have everything as nice as possible for them. If anybody needs pleasant surroundings, who needs them as much as sick people?"[2]

Even in its nascent, pre-Kaiser Permanente form, the innovative mindset of disregarding and disrupting the status quo by understanding and investing in holistic healing was evident.

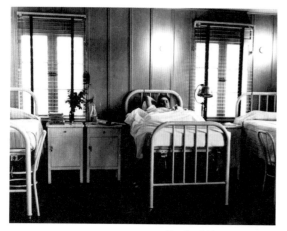

Dr. Garfield was convinced that patients needed an attractive and comfortable environment.

Even in its nascent, pre-Kaiser Permanente form, the innovative mindset of disregarding and disrupting the status quo by understanding and investing in holistic healing was evident.

Runyen soon fell into the work routine. Mornings might include admitting one or two workers for a nonurgent examination and treatment. There was also a steady stream of more serious injuries, mostly fractures and burns. Garfield seemed to be a born teacher. As he treated each patient, he explained what he was doing and why. Runyen found she was learning a great deal more than she had been taught during her three years in nursing school. This on-the-job training was essential because, with a medical staff of only two, Runyen had to perform emergency medical procedures when Garfield was away from the hospital. Once, a patient with heatstroke appeared during such an occurrence, and she started an IV with saline solution. The patient had completely recovered by the time Garfield returned, and he complimented her for her judgment and work.

INNOVATION IN HEALTH CARE FINANCING

The medical side of the hospital operation functioned well, but its operational financing was less certain. Workmen's compensation covered construction workers' health insurance paid by their contractors' insurance companies, and it formed the hospital's economic foundation. After treating a patient, Garfield submitted an itemized report detailing the care provided. At the underwriters' offices, clerks reviewed these reports, disallowing charges they judged were for unnecessary treatment. Although both doctor and nurse provided care, workmen's compensation discounted hospital bills to such a degree that income was not meeting expenses. Garfield was forced to announce to his staff of three and to the underwriters that he was going to have to close down the hospital.

Even though Runyen and the Corbetts were willing to continue working for no salary, just room and board, it still wasn't enough to keep the hospital open.

The Industrial Indemnity Company was the largest underwriter on the Colorado River Aqueduct project. The company realized that closing Contractors General Hospital would mean having to transfer injured workers by ambulance at least to Indio, which was 50 miles across the desert, or to Los Angeles, 130 miles away. This added distance would increase morbidity and mortality as well as expenses. With the goal of keeping the hospital functioning, Harold Hatch, a vice president of Industrial Indemnity, made a simple suggestion that would resonate to the present day.

It illustrated the ingenuity of the time and the value of bold leadership, as he suggested challenging the status quo with an innovative solution that ultimately would transform the economic model of health care delivery.

He suggested that instead of paying Contractors General Hospital for each treatment using the nearly universally accepted fee-for-service model, Industrial Indemnity would prepay Garfield 5 cents a day for each worker covered by the company. So, for the cost of a cup of coffee or candy bar, Garfield and Contractors General would provide whatever medical care the doctor found necessary. The insurance company liked the idea because it would allow them to forecast their medical costs. For his part, Garfield no longer would have the insurance company looking over his shoulder telling him how he should practice medicine.

Also, such a change would mean he would be able to budget based on a known income. Garfield accepted the offer and Hatch helped to convince the other underwriters to join in.

It immediately became evident to Garfield that this capitated 5-cents-a-day model turned the economics of health care upside down. There was now a powerful incentive for him to keep

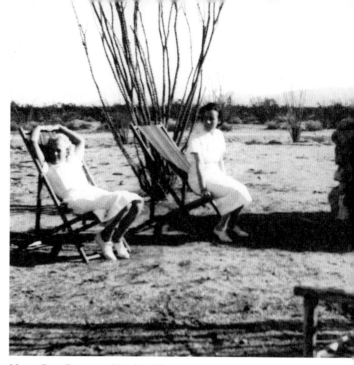

Nurses Betty Runyen and Nadine Cherry enjoy a cool desert evening behind the hospital.

———— • ————

The emergence of this novel, prepaid, wellness-focused approach to health care delivery challenged the dominant sick care model of treatment and its fundamental economic model. This is a classic example of the Kaiser model of seeing opportunity and seizing an innovative solution that introduced entirely new and value-added concepts to health care.

people from needing the hospital's services. It was healthy people, not the sick and injured, who would support the hospital. That nickel per day would change the way physicians, nurses and the medical staff would practice medical care.

The emergence of this novel, prepaid, wellness-focused approach to health care delivery challenged the dominant sick care model of treatment and its fundamental economic model. This is a classic example of the Kaiser model: seeing opportunity and seizing an innovative solution that introduced entirely new and value added concepts to health care.

THE ORIGINS OF THE THRIVE MOTTO: Community-based health promotion and education

Garfield and Runyen began visiting work camps along the aqueduct promoting safety, teaching first aid and encouraging the use of safety equipment. They even set up awards for injury-free work camps. This concern for the maintenance of workers' health would evolve into the *Thrive* motto of Kaiser Permanente decades later and, appropriately, under prepayment, the new hospital did thrive. Garfield invested the money saved through prevention into two new hospitals, several first aid stations and the people to staff them. This gave him the professional satisfaction of knowing that when workers needed care, his facilities now were more accessible. He turned to Runyen to set up and run hospitals or first aid stations. She demonstrated to the new hires what she and Garfield had learned about practicing medicine in a prepaid setting. The staff not only was expected to treat the injuries and illnesses and prescribe treatment, they also were expected to teach their patients how to stay healthy and uninjured while working in a less-than-hospitable part of the country.

The Contractors General Hospitals were not the first to operate under a capitation or prepayment system. The small number of hospitals scattered across the United States that were using a capitation financing system already had drawn the unwelcome attention of the American Medical Association

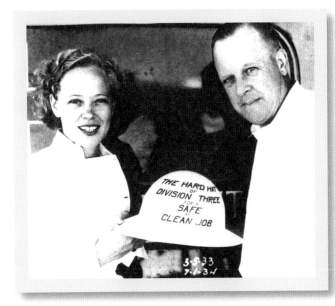

(AMA), which regarded prepayment with suspicion and outright hostility. The AMA claimed the capitation model interfered with the relationship between the patient and physician, and restricted patient choice only to doctors in that particular program.

Nurse Runyen presents safety award. Dr. Garfield immediately understood that prepayment meant an emphasis on prevention.

The Committee on the Costs of Medical Care[3]

The Committee on the Costs of Medical Care (CCMC) was a blue-ribbon group made up of medical economists, physicians in private practice, representatives of medical schools, dentists, nurses and hospitals insurance companies — in short, every stakeholder group in the American health care system. The group's report concluded that **for millions of Americans, the fee-for-service system was not working.** While hospitals and physicians were able to treat more and more conditions, the cost of that care was rising rapidly, putting it out of the reach of millions of families. Rising costs were changing hospital economics. They no longer could rely on philanthropy to finance hospital operations. Unemployment, poverty and the continuing influx of immigrants led to a rapidly increasing number of indigent sick demanding care. Meanwhile, hospital charges and doctor fees were increasing so rapidly that middle-income American families were being priced out of needed health care, and now the Depression was making an already bad situation worse. After a five-year study on the organization, financing and distribution of medical care — and nearly simultaneous to the Contractors General Hospitals' change in financing — the CCMC released its report. Among the recommendations of the majority on this panel were:

- Basic public health services should be extended to the entire population.
- Comprehensive medical care should be provided, preferably by groups of practitioners, organized around hospitals.
- Medical costs should be funded on a group payment basis through insurance premiums, taxation, or both. Fee-for-service care should be available for those who prefer it.
- Professional education should be improved for physicians, health officers, dentists, pharmacists, nurses, nursing aides, midwives, and hospital and clinic administrators.

Today this sounds much like a description of Kaiser Permanente, but in 1932, to most of the medical establishment, this report seemed to strike at the ethical and economic foundations of fee-for-service medicine. The Journal of the American Medical Association went so far as to call the report, "an incitement to revolution."[4] Even if Garfield had been aware of the findings of the CCMC, he would not have been able to see the years of struggle with the AMA that lay ahead of him and Kaiser Permanente about these same issues.

By any measurement, financial or professional, Garfield's desert hospitals were a major success. With an assured income from prepayment, he'd been able to attract well-trained physicians and nurses, and build and operate additional modern and comfortable hospitals and first aid stations even in this remote area. This modest medical practice was too far out of the way to attract unwanted attention, even from an AMA already sensitized by the Committee on the Costs of Medical Care (CCMC) to the possible challenge posed by group practice funded by prepayment. However, it was clear that the AMA's virulent opposition to the principle of prepaid group practice made it highly unlikely Garfield would have a chance to develop his concepts further.

THE GROWTH OF HENRY J. KAISER'S INDUSTRIAL PROJECTS AND THE IMPACT ON HEALTH CARE DELIVERY

At the same time that work on the Southern California aqueduct was nearing completion, Henry J. Kaiser and his partners, doing business as Six Companies Inc., were preparing to carry out a contract to build a gigantic dam across the nearly mile wide Columbia River in eastern Washington state, employing 5,000 workers.

The various entities of Six Companies already had some impressive projects under their collective belt, including the Hoover, Parker and Bonneville Dams, all successfully completed ahead of schedule and under budget. However, there was a potential problem at Grand Coulee. Under the previous contractor, workers had completed the first phase, the dam's foundation, but those workers had been very dissatisfied with the medical care that had been available. They demanded that their union, and not the Kaiser group, run the new medical care program. Kaiser and his partners did not agree, but recognized that something had to be done to reassure workers that the Six Companies would provide quality care. The search for a better way led to young Dr. Garfield and his prepaid medical practice ideas.

Grand Coulee Dam, as big as it was, was just one of Henry Kaiser's projects. The actual head of the dam construction was his son, Edgar Kaiser. Edgar Kaiser's obvious determination to provide quality health care to the workers convinced an originally reluctant Garfield to take on the job, applying what he had learned in the California desert to a program where the workers were all in one area, rather than being stretched out as they had been along the aqueduct.

Once he agreed to take the job, the young surgeon began work on two fronts — renovating the existing ill-equipped and run-down hospital that already existed at the dam site, and recruiting a medical staff to this remote site in eastern Washington.

With the help of Edgar Kaiser, the hospital renovation went well, with Garfield insisting that it be well equipped and also attractive and comfortable for patients. However, finding physicians willing to move to this isolated worksite proved more difficult than he had expected.

The first of the physicians to sign on was Wallace "Wally" Neighbor, a Washington native and a close Garfield friend going back to their days as medical residents at Los Angeles County Hospital. However, getting others to move to a small town in the high desert of Eastern Washington turned out to be quite frustrating. His luck turned when he convinced Cecil Cutting, a Stanford graduate and surgical resident at San Francisco General Hospital, to join him. Cutting was so respected by

his colleagues that his enthusiasm for the Coulee Dam project convinced two Stanford classmates, Ray Gillette and Richard Moore, to join him. Meanwhile, Garfield succeeded in hiring Gene Wiley, a classmate from his days at the University of Iowa's medical school. Together, they formed the hospital staff which was named Sidney Garfield and Associates.

The nursing staff was taking shape, too. Cecil Cutting's wife, Millie, a nurse at San Francisco General Hospital, brought her friend, Winnie Wetherill (who would marry Wally Neighbor; their daughter, Nelle, was the first baby to be born in a Kaiser hospital), also from San Francisco General. Both of them joined Isabel Moore and Hazel Gillette, Millie's classmates at Stanford nursing school.

————— • —————

They were unaware they were pioneering a model of team-based care delivery decades before its efficacy would be understood as a best practices model of care.

——————————

When a patient died on the operating table, Cutting thought the patient might have survived if there had been an anesthesia specialist in the operating room. Cutting asked Geraldine Searcy, a nurse anesthetist who had spent the previous two years working with him at San Francisco General, to join the Coulee group.

The young staff of this medical outpost were bound together by interlocking friendships, the dam's remoteness, and professional respect based on their experience with one another. They spent their free time at Grand Coulee picnicking, horse-back riding, fishing and attending parties. For most of them it was one of the most enjoyable times of their lives, both personally and professionally.[5]

They were unaware they were pioneering a model of team-based care delivery decades before its efficacy would be understood as a best practices model of care.

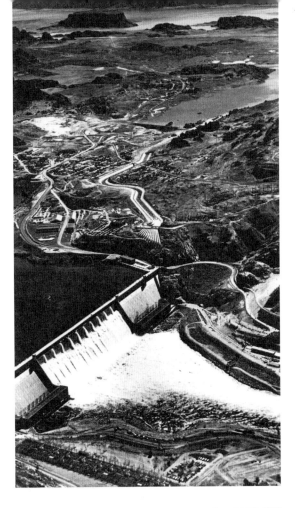

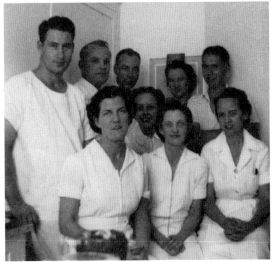

(Top to bottom) Nearly a mile across, Grand Coulee Dam was called "The Mightiest Thing Ever built by a Man" c. 1940.

Physicians and nurses pose for photograph – Mason City Hospital at Grand Coulee Dam site c. 1938.

CAPITATION AND THE COST SAVINGS OF PREVENTIVE CARE

As in the Mojave Desert, the Coulee program was based on prepayment by workmen's compensation underwriters that covered work-related injuries and illnesses. For an additional voluntary 50 cents a week, Garfield offered the workers prepaid comprehensive coverage. However, their wives and children still received medical care on a fee-for-service basis. Before long, the group noticed that fee-for-service patients were delaying medical care until their symptoms were severe, while prepaid patients came earlier, when their illnesses were easier to treat effectively. The workers noticed this, too, and soon were demanding that their families have the same coverage they were receiving. There was even talk of a strike if such coverage couldn't be arranged.

Once the families were enrolled in prepaid coverage, the staff began seeing patients sooner in their illnesses' progression — before bronchitis had turned into potentially fatal pneumonia, and before those with diabetes went into crisis. Staff were treating inflamed appendixes rather than ruptured ones. Garfield saw that "with the barrier of cost removed, people were coming into us earlier in their illnesses, before it was too late to do anything about it." He later said of this time, simply, "People stopped dying."[6]

Garfield later said he and his medical staff also felt a responsibility toward the general community.[7] Physician and nurse volunteers established and ran education programs, as well as a well-baby clinic headed by Millie Cutting.

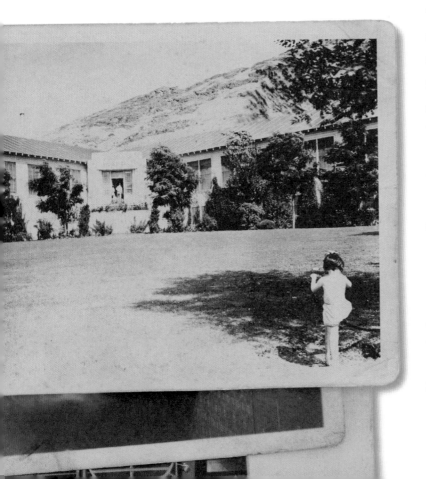

Hospital at Mason City,
Washington c. 1938.

Now caring for 15,000 workers and family members, Garfield hired additional specialists, including a pediatrician and an obstetrician/gynecologist. This no longer was industrial medicine: he now was running a full-service medical program. Its hallmarks included prepayment, prevention, group practice, and integrated hospital-based care.

THE RESHAPING OF AMERICAN MEDICINE

It was at Grand Coulee that Garfield first met Edgar's father, Henry Kaiser. In their first conversation, the 56-year-old industrialist warmed to the young physician and immediately grasped the potential of Garfield's approach to health care. Kaiser told him, "Young man, if your idea is half as good as you say it is, it is good for the entire country."[8] Their resulting friendship soon would reshape American medicine. As Garfield later would say of the Grand Coulee experience, it was "the final dress rehearsal" for what would become Kaiser Permanente.[9]

In early 1941, almost a year before the attack on Pearl Harbor, Henry Kaiser had realized there soon would be a huge demand for new ships. A businessman always on the lookout for new business opportunities, Kaiser now expanded his activities into shipbuilding and built a shipyard in Richmond, California. This was the beginning of an explosive period of growth for Kaiser's business operations. Within a month of the attack on Pearl Harbor, there already were two Kaiser shipyards in operation, another just beginning construction and yet another scheduled to start in June. The workforce, already at 30,000, was expected to rise rapidly to 90,000 in Richmond alone. Overall, Kaiser's workforce in the shipyards and in support of that work rose to nearly 200,000 on the West Coast, including three Kaiser shipyards in the Vancouver, Washington area and his steel mill in Fontana, in southern California.

As workers from all over America poured into the shipyards, a shortage of medical care became a critical issue affecting worker morale and therefore production. Kaiser workers who had transferred from Grand Coulee were grumbling that they were not getting the kind of medical care they had become accustomed to, and they resented it.

Medical care was especially important in the shipyards since the able-bodied men had been drafted for military service. Most workers coming to Richmond from around the country had been classified as too old or too unhealthy and physically unfit for military service. Many actually suf-

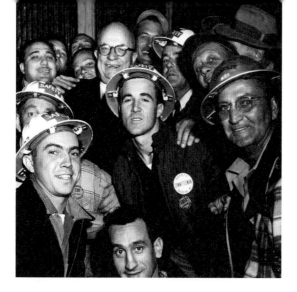

fered from chronic illnesses. Dr. Cutting later would describe the shipyard workers as "a walking pathological museum."[10] In addition, their inexperience in the heavy construction trades led to frequent accidents and high illness rates.

THE KAISERS TURN TO GARFIELD AGAIN

As the dam at Grand Coulee neared completion, Garfield had returned to Los Angeles to teach surgery at the University of Southern California medical school. When Henry Kaiser Jr., the 24-year-old son of Henry Kaiser, reached out to him to set up a medical care program for the rapidly expanding shipyards, he learned that Dr. Garfield had enlisted in the University of Southern California's U.S. Army Medical Corps and was scheduled to leave for India the next month. Henry Kaiser Jr., who was focusing on personnel issues, convinced Garfield to, at a minimum, visit the shipyards as a medical systems consultant before shipping out. He could at least design, if not run, a new shipyard medical program.

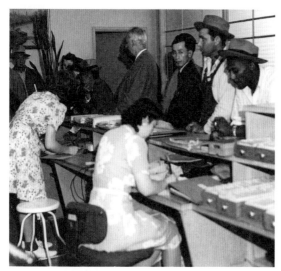

(Top to bottom) A jovial Henry Kaiser surrounded by happy shipyard workers. Front desk at the Richmond Field Hospital. Aerial view of ship launching at Richmond Shipyard.

(Opposite left to right) First Aid station RN with young worker in chair. President Roosevelt visits Henry J. Kaiser for launch of the SS Joseph Teal Sept. 23, 1942. Former Fabiola Hospital, keystone of Permanente Health Plan; Dedication Day, August 21, 1942.

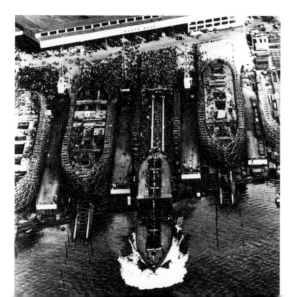

THE WAR EFFORT, BIRTH OF OAKLAND MEDICAL CENTER AND WHAT WOULD BECOME THE FUTURE SITE OF THE KAISER FOUNDATION SCHOOL OF NURSING

It didn't take long for the Kaisers to realize Garfield was the only person who could run the new shipyard health plan. Henry Kaiser Sr. sent a request directly to President Roosevelt, who released Garfield from the Army to facilitate the production of ships desperately needed to carry on a two-ocean war against Germany and Japan.[11]

Now released from the Army, Garfield's first order of business was to find, equip and open a hospital that would be the centerpiece of the new medical program in the shipyards. The best candidate for the role was what remained of the defunct and abandoned four-story Fabiola Hospital — formerly a 50-bed maternity hospital — on the corner of Broadway and Moss Avenue in Oakland.[12] The hospital was 12 miles from the shipyards, but emergency care could be provided at the smaller field hospital, which was under construction and much closer to the shipyards on Cutting Boulevard. The plan was that after an emergency patient was stabilized, he would be transported to the Kaiser's Fabiola Hospital in Oakland.

The Fabiola Hospital was owned by Samuel Merritt Hospital, which had no plans for it. The concrete building already had been partially torn down. Many of the inside partitions had been ripped out,

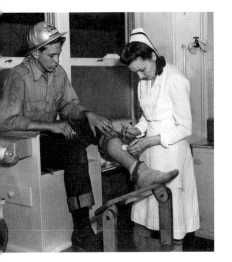
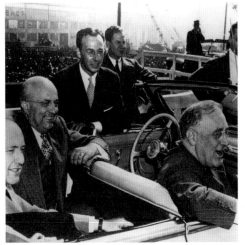
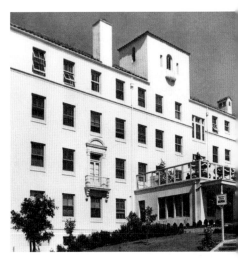

and floors were covered with broken pipes and rubble. With a $250,000 Bank of America loan guaranteed by Henry Kaiser, Garfield had his hospital.

Although he was a surgeon, Garfield had wanted to be an architect, and throughout his medical training and practice, he had been developing ideas that would make hospitals more efficient and safer. With Kaiser's support, Garfield transformed the abandoned hulk of a building into a first-class hospital ready for patients in less than six months. This extraordinary burst of effort, innovation and achievement was accomplished despite major wartime shortages.

While the new hospital was being built, Garfield had arranged for patients to be treated at local hospitals. By the day of the official opening on Aug. 21, 1942, those patients already had been moved into the new building. Nurse anesthetist Gerry Searcy remembered the opening. She recalled that although the staff was busy with patients, some of them were able to rush outside to spend a few minutes at the celebration.[13] They heard Henry Kaiser dedicate the building to the memory of his mother, who had died prematurely at age 52 from a lack of access to proper medical care.

In addition to the Fabiola Hospital, Garfield had another major project. In February, the United States Maritime Commission, overseer of the shipyard activities, began building a small field hospital in Richmond on Cutting Avenue not far from the yards. The new hospital would provide immediate care to the injured and, when they were stabilized, send them by ambulance to the main hospital in Oakland. Dr. Garfield's medical staff would be operating the facility. Garfield had the opportunity to apply his innovative ideas in hospital design to this new building.

While setting up the shipyard health plan, Garfield had realized that if it were possible to operate it as a nonprofit foundation, he might be able to redirect tax savings to fund the program's continuing operations in the postwar world.

This way of thinking and seeing obstacles as opportunities exposed a completely new avenue for structuring health care financing that would influence modern health care economic structures. Innovation followed by courageous leadership and action marked these early days of what would become Kaiser Permanente.

At Grand Coulee, he and many of the Coulee staff had talked about moving the program to an urban setting after the dam was completed, but nothing had come from that. The hostility of organized medicine seemed to be an insurmountable barrier. Now that they were already established in Richmond, a postwar program seemed like a real possibility. However, he would need help from Henry Kaiser to make this a reality.

———— • ————

This way of thinking and seeing obstacles as opportunities exposed a completely new avenue for structuring health care financing that would influence modern health care economic structures. Innovation followed by courageous leadership and action marked these early days of what would become Kaiser Permanente.

————————

Getting time with the busy industrialist to explain his unusual idea for funding such a program was difficult, but Garfield managed to get two uninterrupted hours with Kaiser by going to Sacramento and boarding the train to Oakland to accompany the industrialist on the final leg of a return trip from Washington, D.C. Garfield explained to Kaiser his thoughts on how they might start a tax-free foundation that would fund itself. This was a highly unusual concept. Foundations such as those of Ford and Rockefeller and many others almost always were funded by major bequests. Kaiser's lawyers gave many reasons why this could not and should not be done. Kaiser, who already had learned at Grand Coulee to appreciate the power and efficiency of a medical care program based on prepayment, snapped, "I'm sick and tired of having lawyers tell me things we can't do. Now you tell me how we can do it. That's your job."[14]

The attorneys did find a way. They founded the nonprofit Permanente Foundation, which became the new owner of the Fabiola Hospital, renamed Permanente Hospital. The Permanente Health Plan was now nonprofit, and as Garfield had foreseen, the assets of the new foundation began to grow.

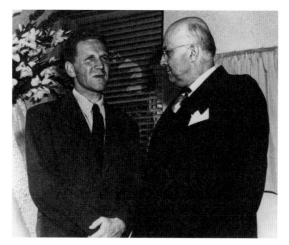

Garfield and Kaiser confer during dedication of the new Permanente Hospital, August 21, 1942.

The core of the new hospital's staff was the nurses and doctors who had been with Garfield at Coulee. They brought with them a sense of camaraderie and collegiality that had been developed during their Grand Coulee years, which would help shape the attitudes and working relationships in Oakland. These were men and women who already were familiar with Garfield's vision and were committed to it. As Garfield often pointed out, other insurance plans were, in reality, sick plans, profiting from illness and injury. They were building what would be a true health plan based not only on healing the sick and injured, but also on preserving health by involving patient/members in their own care through education and prevention.

The shipyard newspaper, Fore 'N' Aft, became a part of the health program. It carried regular health and accident prevention features. Fore 'N' Aft described the new health plan's primary goal as "the prevention of illness through medical treatment administered at the proper time." There were articles about a women's breast and uterine cancer detection clinic for the growing number of female workers. Luncheon entertainment broadcasts over the shipyard loudspeaker also carried nutrition information, tips on how to avoid colds, encouraged daily exercise and offered safety tips.

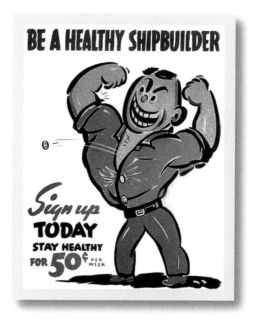

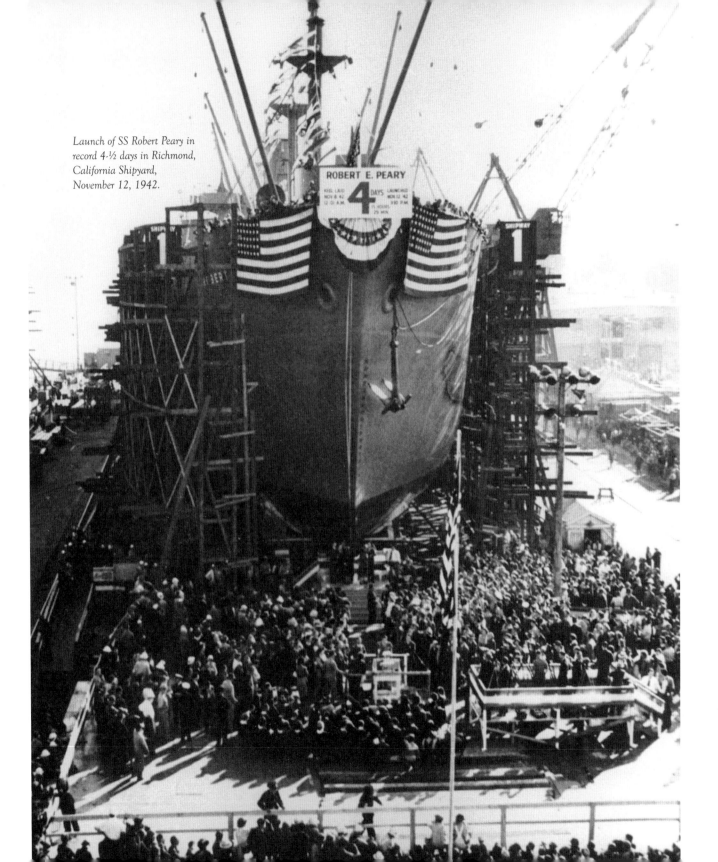

Launch of SS Robert Peary in record 4-½ days in Richmond, California Shipyard, November 12, 1942.

MEASURABLE RESULTS: A RECORD OF ON-THE-JOB
SAFETY AND COMMUNITY, WELLNESS-BASED CARE

Soon there was good reason to think the program's emphasis on prevention was working. On July 30, 1942, the United States Maritime Commission, the government agency in charge of the shipbuilding program, cited Kaiser's Richmond yards for an outstanding record for on-the-job safety. It had the lowest loss ratio due to injuries and illnesses and the lowest time loss of productive manhours of any wartime industry in California. This was particularly impressive since the majority of the shipyard workers had no experience in heavy construction.

To treat injured workers, Garfield set up six first aid stations at key locations within the shipyards and staffed them with his physicians and nurses. Rae Englemann, a nurse anesthetist who had been at Grand Coulee, described the treatment process. "If someone was injured at the shipyard, they'd be treated at the first aid station and then they'd be sent to the Field Hospital for evaluation – should they be sent home or shipped to Oakland. It was almost like a MASH unit."[15]

Harriet Stewart, a young nurse from Nebraska who began her nearly 40-year Kaiser career in a Kaiser shipyard first aid station before women were hired in the shipyard workforce, recalled, "We were the only women allowed in the shipyard, and we had respect like you wouldn't believe. We wore nurses' uniforms, nurses' hats, white shoes, and we conducted ourselves like we were taught in training – you know, as ladies." She also remembered an important feature built into the medical care program right from the beginning: "There was no discrimination of any sort in our care. If (African American workers) were sick and they needed care, they were given the care that the white men were given, and with respect."[16]

Workers with more serious injuries were taken by shipyard station wagons directly to the nearby field hospital. Those needing more care were transported a few miles away to Oakland and the thoroughly modernized Permanente Hospital.

Another nurse, Millie Cutting, had come to the shipyards from Grand Coulee with her husband, surgeon Cecil Cutting. She became an unofficial and very effective purchasing agent for the program. Using a shipyard station wagon, she scoured the Bay Area, warehouses and drugstores for the scarce supplies needed to keep the program running.

By late 1944, it was clear that the war was moving toward a victorious end. Although no one could predict when it would be over, the sense of crisis that had mobilized the American public and industries since Pearl Harbor was easing. Henry Kaiser's Richmond shipyards cut back the 24/7 schedule to six days. Layoffs reduced the workforce from 90,000 to 65,000. For Garfield's staff, it was a look into their future — and it was bleak. The income from dues necessary to remain in operation was dropping and likely would continue to drop unless something could be done. Then, suddenly, atomic bombs exploded over Nagasaki and Hiroshima. The war was over and soon the worker rolls were down to 10,000.

On a positive note, the Kaiser Foundation Health Plan, operating as the nonprofit Permanente Foundation, had matured into a prepaid group practice whose hallmarks included illness prevention and hospital-based integrated services.

Many of the physicians and nurses began retiring or moving back to their hometown practices. But for a handful of physicians, 13 out of the nearly 100 who had made up Sidney Garfield and Associates during the war, the possibility of opening up the program to the public and keeping the health plan going seemed both possible and very desirable.

It was with this sense of mission and the belief that the program they had developed was worth saving that the remaining staff prepared to make the sacrifices needed to shift the foundation from a wartime footing to a community-based health plan. This would soon include a school of nursing.

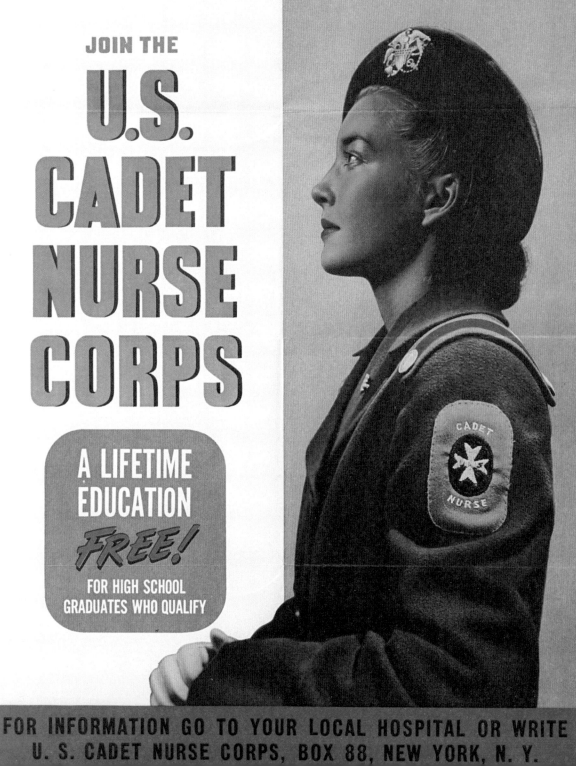

MODEL *of* INNOVATION

ENDURING LEGACIES ② IN NURSING EDUCATION

The Birth of the Kaiser Foundation School of Nursing

WORLD WAR II'S INFLUENCE ON THE FOUNDING OF THE SCHOOL OF NURSING To find the roots of nursing education at Kaiser Permanente, you need to look deep into its history. In August 1942, at the dedication of what would become the first hospital in the Kaiser Permanente system, Henry Kaiser outlined four goals for the new Permanente Foundation. Among them was to "set up fellowships for the training of physicians and nurses in specialties."[1]

This was a clear commitment to medical education. It also implied that physicians and nurses not only would train together, but that they would be trained in medical specialties. This was a new and radical idea in nursing education. In 1944, Dr. Sidney Garfield moved toward that goal. He committed The Permanente Foundation Health Plan, precursor to the Kaiser Health Plan, to nursing education by the formal notification to the California Board of Nursing Examiners that he was planning to establish a three-year diploma school of nursing in Oakland. In Garfield's second annual report to The Permanente Foundation in 1945, he wrote, "We are planning an accredited school of nursing which will be free from the traditional pressure of economics on nursing education, and permit proper emphasis and time in the purely medical aspects of instruction, carrying this on to nursing specialization in the various fields and medical care on a parallel with resident physician training in medicine."[2]

During negotiations for the proposed school, the Board of Nurse Examiners (now known as the California Board of Registered Nurses) asked whether the newly formed United States Cadet

*Applying the Cadet Corps'
approach to diversity and
use of stipends at a private
school showed an openness
to innovation and courage to
try bold new approaches that
would come to exemplify the
culture and leadership of
modern-day Kaiser Permanente.*

Nurse Corps could place its senior students at the Permanente Foundation Hospital in Oakland for the clinical practice part of their education. Garfield agreed.

The U.S. Cadet Nurse Corps, operating under the supervision of the U.S. Public Health Service, had been formed in July 1943 to relieve the acute shortage of military and civilian nurses through an accelerated program.

There were startling resemblances between the U.S. Cadet Corps and the soon-to-be organized Permanente School of Nursing.[3] The cadet program was open to high school graduates and young women of all ethnicities. Surprisingly, this included Japanese American women who had been interned in the relocation camps set up shortly after the attack on Pearl Harbor in December 1941; they were released in order to serve as military nurses.[4] A federal subsidy paid for students' tuition, room, uniforms, board and a small stipend. Garfield later would adopt this policy at his nursing school.

Applying the Cadet Corps' approach to diversity and use of stipends at a private school showed an openness to innovation and courage to try bold new approaches that would come to exemplify the culture and leadership of modern-day Kaiser Permanente. The cadets were assigned to support the Kaiser Fabiola Hospital nursing staff; they had a major role in relieving the hospital's wartime nursing shortage. Throughout the remainder of World War II, Permanente's arrangement with the Cadet Nurse Corps worked well for both the corps and for Permanente.

To Garfield, the cadet nurse experience had far greater implications than merely solving a personnel shortage. The experience also served as a kind of dress rehearsal for a nursing school of his own.

He recognized that the students had been "a great stimulus to our professional staff." In the January 1945 issue of the Permanente Bulletin, he wrote: "The organization of this training program for cadet nurses and our intern-resident program ... appears to be one of the most outstanding achievements of the year."[5]

Significantly, in the Bulletin article, he had linked the advantages of integrating the cadet nurses' training with Permanente's intern-resident program.

POST-WORLD WAR II: ECONOMICS AND EMPLOYMENT SHAPE NURSING NEEDS AND A RESPONSE TO THE HEALTH PLAN

Immediately after World War II, Garfield and the medical program faced a new set of challenges. As the shipyards shut down, dues-paying workers left to find other jobs. Health Plan income plummeted by more than 90 percent. Most of the medical staff in Oakland were there only for the duration of the war; many returned to their private practices or retired.

The medical program, so successful while the shipyards were operating at full strength, now was hanging on by a thread. Faced with the problem of continuing to finance operations as the shipyards shut down, Garfield roamed through the organization looking for ways to cut overhead. Perhaps the best-remembered of his efforts is The Pencil Stub Club.

The Pencil Stub Club grew out of Garfield's attempt to control office expenses by requiring employees to turn in the stub of a pencil in order to get a new, full-length one. The pencil stub idea was one of a number of cost-cutting procedures he put into effect, and one of the smallest, but it was symbolic of his efforts to make the staff cost conscious. In 1983, the Pencil Stub Club was formed to honor those long-time employees who had helped the Health Plan survive by holding down the costs of running Kaiser Permanente. The club helped commemorate and perpetuate Garfield's conviction that to every extent possible, member dues ought to be applied to member care.[6]

A while after the shipyards closed, membership rolls began to grow again as a number of union workers in the rapidly growing Bay Area started demanding the kind of medical coverage they'd had when working in the Kaiser shipyards. During this period, the IRS ruled that insurance benefits no longer would be treated as income. This meant that health insurance could become a tax-free benefit to be negotiated by unions with employers. That feature, and word-of-mouth recommendations based on member satisfaction, fueled rapid postwar membership growth.

While membership growth certainly was welcome, it brought new challenges. Most significantly, local physicians were beginning to see the Health Plan as a major economic threat, and they began to fight back. In a campaign of rumor, innuendo and deliberate misinformation, the Alameda-Contra Costa Medical Society, supported by the American Medical Association, began spreading rumors that Henry Kaiser controlled the program and that Health Plan "profits" were going into his pocket. They even claimed the program was "socialized medicine," which it clearly was not, but the post-

war period was a time when terms like "socialized medicine" were thrown about thoughtlessly but effectively in an attempt to make the Health Plan appear "un-American," thus making it difficult for the emerging medical group. Permanente physicians were not even allowed to join the local medical society.[7]

Although the fee-for-service physicians charged the Health Plan and the Permanente physicians with ethical violations and practicing "socialized medicine," at the heart of the dispute was that the Health Plan was providing economic competition and the AMA and medical societies wanted to crush it before it became more of a threat to physician income.

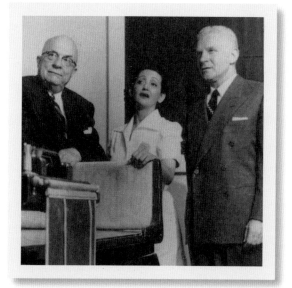

Henry Kaiser (left) with Dorothea Daniels and Sidney Garfield inspecting a new x-ray machine at the Oakland Hospital.

For Garfield and Henry Kaiser, this was one of the countless times where adversity became the mother of invention.

Professional hostility lead to making it difficult for the program to recruit the nurses and physicians they needed to care for their growing membership. Worse still, this eventually could affect quality of care. Despite predictions to the contrary, war's end had not brought an end to the national nursing shortage, since many military nurses chose to retire from nursing rather than go into civilian practice upon returning home.

These problems, along with the experience the Permanente Foundation Hospital already had with the Cadet Nurse Corps, made a strong case that it was time for the medical program to begin training its own nurses.

For Garfield and Henry Kaiser, this was one of the countless times where adversity became the mother of invention.

In June 1947, with approval from the California Board of Nursing Examiners, the Permanente School of Nursing began "… preparing young women in the art and science of nursing with special emphasis to be placed on the teachings of methods of protecting community health and on the skills and techniques of bedside nursing."[8]

The nursing school needed to affiliate with a college where students could take the basic science courses they needed for their training. The College of the Holy Names was selected for this role. Students also could take general education classes, which they could apply toward a bachelor's degree. From the beginning, there was an expectation that many students would continue their education to receive a college degree after receiving their RN training.

As the opening date for the new school drew nearer, there was an all-out push to find students. At the time, the traditional career choices for women, along with nursing, were secretary and teacher. The Permanente School of Nursing provided an appealing option. Not only was there no tuition, which was common among nursing schools at the time, the Permanente School of Nursing also offered free room, board, books,

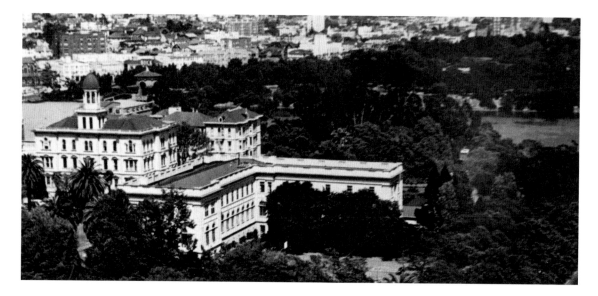

uniforms and even a stipend. This made the school particularly attractive to minorities and students from families who otherwise could not afford to send a daughter to nursing school. Furthermore, enrollment was open to all, including Japanese American and African American students. It was an attractive opportunity.

The nondiscriminatory policy was rooted in earlier Kaiser organizations and was already a part of the Kaiser organizational culture. Avram Yedidia, a health care economist who had begun his career with Kaiser in the wartime shipyards, was interviewed by the University of California's Bancroft Library in a series of oral histories preserving California history.

"I recall one day, probably in 1946, when the chief of police of Oakland, along with his top staff, came to visit the hospital to see what we were doing, with the view that maybe some of them would like to join the health plan. I recall that we were standing on a deck next to the surgical suite looking over MacArthur Boulevard. And the police chief said to me, 'You know, when we walked through, I saw that you had some Negroes and whites in the same room. I don't think we like that.'"

The implication was that if the Health Plan did not change its policy, the department would not sign up. Despite the need for income, Yedidia, who often was called "the social conscience of

Kaiser Permanente," said, "Those who don't like it shouldn't join the plan."[9]

Yedidia also recounted another story that had been passed around the Health Plan and made clear Henry Kaiser's thinking about discrimination. "He [Kaiser] was asked, 'Should we really separate our patients? After all, we only have two beds in each place,[10] and so it would be easy to manage it.' He scratched his bald head, so I was told, and he said, 'You know, if I were a black man, and you were going to put me along with everybody like me on the right side of the hall, and you had gold carpets there, and there was that miserable tile that I told you not to put in on the left side of the hall where the whites were placed, I still wouldn't believe that you treated me equally.'"

Embracing diversity and subsidizing educational costs were building blocks for the Kaiser Foundation School of Nursing, the early hallmarks and emerging legacy of what became Kaiser Permanente's longstanding approach of disrupting the status quo of nursing education.

What makes both of these statements remarkable is that they were made at a time when every private hospital in the San Francisco Bay Area was segregated, and the Health Plan was desperately seeking new members to replace the tens of thousands lost after WWII. Even so, considerations of social justice prevailed over the need for new members.

(Opposite) College of the Holy Names (Holy Names College) beside Lake Merritt, future site of the Kaiser Center.

All patients were treated the same. There was no discrimination in the Kaiser world.

Embracing diversity and subsidizing educational costs were building blocks for the Kaiser Foundation School of Nursing, the early hallmarks and emerging legacy of what became Kaiser Permanente's long-standing approach of disrupting the status quo of nursing education.

RECRUITING THE FIRST CLASS OF THE PERMANENTE SCHOOL OF NURSING

Recruitment of students was intense and varied. Information about the school was sent to high school teachers, school nurses and high school nursing clubs throughout northern and central California. The school even advertised in newspapers. A newspaper was how Francine Weir Ammerman, a member of the charter class of 1950, first learned about the school.

"There was a tiny little thing in the ad section. They were recruiting young girls to be a part of it. We spent our first six months in Vallejo at a facility that I think had been military at one time. We were each assigned a room. The first day, we had a watermelon feed in the back yard where we all got to know each other. It all started right then and there. Some of my classmates didn't remember that but I did. There were no table[s] or chairs, a lot of weeds and high grass back there, but they chopped up a bunch of watermelons and we all ate watermelon and got to know each other a little bit."[11, 12]

SCHOOL STARTUP: THE EARLY MONTHS

At first, school personnel consisted only of the director of nursing at the Permanente Hospital, Clare Wangen, and two instructors, Bea Benson and Maxine Lueck.[13] Wangen also was the founding director of the school and she selected students for that first class. Later, as the faculty expanded, the director formed a small admissions committee that sought young women with good grades who already had shown an interest in nursing, perhaps through volunteering in a local hospital or as members of their high school's Future Nurse's Club.

The students were mostly 18 years old and from small towns in northern and central California, but there also were students who came to the school from southern California, Colorado, Hawaii, North

Dakota, Samoa and even the East Coast. Often their reason for applying was to get away from home. Since attending nursing school was their first time living independently, these students found the support they received from the faculty and housemothers helped them adjust to the daily challenges of living on their own away from their families.

On Aug. 25, 1947, the Oakland-based nursing school began operations not in Oakland, but in Vallejo, at the former Community Hospital about 25 miles from Oakland. It was only temporary. The Community Hospital had been declared war surplus, so with an eye toward growth The Permanente Foundation purchased it. However, it would take several years for the program to grow into this new facility. Until permanent quarters were found, the unused space became the temporary home of the new school.

Original financial support for the school came from three sources: the Permanente Hospital, The Permanente Foundation and from the Kaiser family.

1948 Dos and Don'ts

The first Permanente School of Nursing student handbook, developed in 1948, prescribed the dos and don'ts for students to get along well at the school:

- Your ability as a nurse is reflected in the way you keep your room.
- Students must be in their own room at 10 p.m., and all lights will be out at 10:30 p.m.
- Guests may be entertained only in the living room between 8 a.m. and 10 p.m. (exceptions were made if a parent came to visit).
- Pre-clinical students will be in the residence at 8 p.m. each day, Monday through Thursday, unless otherwise specified by the director of nurses.
- Your window shades will be kept drawn at night when the lights are on.
- Every student is expected to be adequately clothed when going through the halls.
- Students are expected to be tidy and well-groomed at all times.
- The conduct of the student nurse on and off duty must be such as will not reflect discredit on herself, her chosen profession, nor her school.[14]

Charter Class
Student Handbook.

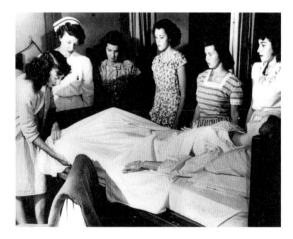

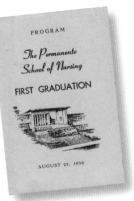

PROGRAM
The Permanente School of Nursing
FIRST GRADUATION

AUGUST 25, 1950

Applicants who had been selected for the first class were instructed to bring a watch with a second hand, a fountain pen and a few of what then were called "wash dresses." These were plain cotton frocks they could wash by hand. The startup had been so quick that the school had no time to order uniforms. Students wore these simple dresses to class and in the wards until their new uniforms arrived.

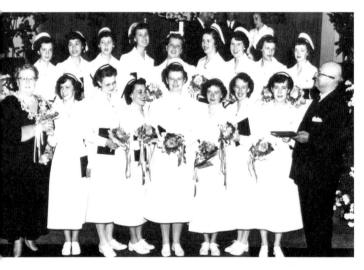

The students learned the most basic nursing skills in their initial classes: how to take a blood pressure, a temperature and a pulse; how to give a bed bath and injections; and how to make a bed with and without a patient in it. Under the watchful eyes of their instructors and with the patients' permission, students were able to apply these new skills on patients rather than merely practice on one another. Classroom work, said student Francine Weir, went "hand in glove with bedside experience."

(Top to bottom) Charter Class students in wash dresses begin training caring for "Mrs. Chase," medical mannequin.

Henry and Bess Kaiser at first graduation.

Henry Kaiser hands diploma to a member of the first graduating class.

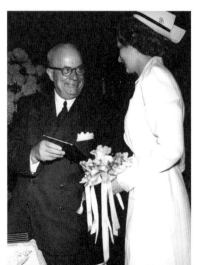

Throughout the next 29 years, the school's "hand in glove" integration of classroom work with bedside experience was a key element in the Permanente approach to nursing education.

Several weeks into that first term, students finally were able to change out of the wash dresses they'd brought from home and wear one of the six attractive blue uniforms with white bibs they'd been issued. Since this class would be the only one to have blue uniforms, subsequent classes gave them the nickname, "The Blue Brats." Other classes were issued uniforms that were light pastel green, Bess Kaiser's favorite color, which became known as Permanente Green. The same color was used to decorate walls in some parts of the hospital. Subsequent classes wore yellow dress uniforms.

Henry Kaiser had a particular interest in the nursing school. On August 3, 1950, the school graduated its first class; a proud Henry and Bess Kaiser attended the graduation, where the industrialist shared his thoughts and appreciation of the nursing profession. He began with a touching story of his mother, Maria, who died in his arms because she didn't have access to good medical care. In his talk to the young women, he did not emphasize why she died — he spoke of how she'd lived and linked that to his admiration of nurses.

What's in a Name?

In 1938, Henry Kaiser expanded into the cement business. He built a plant in the hills above Cupertino on the peninsula south of San Francisco. The area was known as Permanente because of a picturesque stream that continued running through the property year round, even through the dry season. The cement produced there was Kaiser's Permanente Cement, the first time the two names were linked. Bess Kaiser was particularly fond of the Permanente name and it soon became the name of several other Kaiser companies, including the shipyards; the medical care program for the yard workers was known as the Permanente Health Plan.

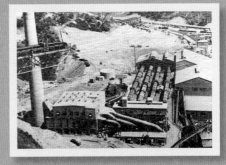

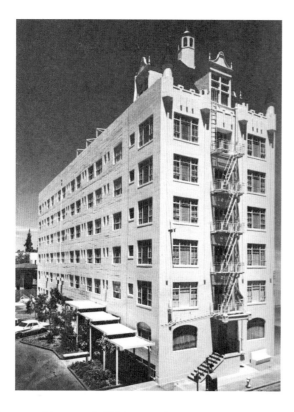

In the graduation speech titled, "The Nurse's Profession of Giving to Mankind" he told the graduates, "One of the Greatest of All Services Rendered to Mankind Is Rendered By Nurses, ... My mother nursed her suffering neighbors. I grew up at a time when there were extremely few trained nurses, and in a community that had only one doctor. One of my most vivid boyhood memories is of my mother, how after working in her own home looking after her own family, would be ready and glad to go out at night to donate her nursing talents to neighbors needing care. ... So the memory of Mother always giving of herself to others has inspired in me a tremendous appreciation of the great work of service and giving carried out by our nurses. ... It is my conviction that the careers of giving and serving which you have dedicated your lives to give you true happiness — the most genuine kind of success and happiness there is on this earth."[15]

Sadly, Bess Kaiser's participation in that first graduation was also her last, but her vigorous support of the endeavor was well-known. When she passed away in early spring 1951 at the age of

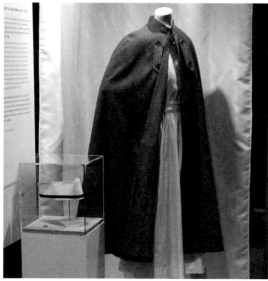

(Top to bottom) Piedmont Hotel, home of the school of nursing.

Nursing student uniform, cap and cape.

65, School Director Dorothea Daniels arranged the farewell tribute — a student honor guard — to a woman who had been an enthusiastic supporter of the school from the very beginning. Two students in uniforms and capes stood at attention in 15-minute shifts beside the casket at the Albert Brown Mortuary directly across the street from the school. Roberta Smith Neary, class of '51A, treasured many keepsakes from her years at KFSN, including a gold charm she described as bearing the image of St. Christopher on one side and on the other the date of Bess Kaiser's death. It was a memento given by Henry Kaiser to each of the young women who had been part of the honor guard.

THE SCHOOL'S NEW LOCATION: FROM VALLEJO TO OAKLAND

For its first few months of operation, the school remained headquartered in Vallejo while Garfield searched for a more suitable location. He found a six-story hotel on Piedmont Avenue, only a short walk from the Oakland hospital, owned by twin brothers named Bass. Since Garfield wasn't sure their price was fair, he turned to the Kaiser Industries organization for help. Henry Kaiser's chief operating officer, Gene Trefethen, sent one of his financial assistants, William Soule, on a Saturday to meet with the brothers, inspect the building, look at their financial ledgers and make a recommendation about the price. Late that afternoon, after careful consideration of all aspects of the building, Soule told Trefethen the price was fair. Trefethen thanked him and said he was glad to hear it because Garfield had been so anxious to have a permanent home for the nursing school he already had made an offer on the building![16] What had been the Piedmont Hotel was now going to be the Permanente School of Nursing.

STAFFING CHANGES: DOROTHEA DANIELS APPOINTED
TO FULFILL GARFIELD'S VISION FOR THE SCHOOL

The appointment of Clare Wangen to be the first director of the Permanente School of Nursing had been a natural one. She had trained at Johns Hopkins Hospital in Baltimore and already was director of nursing at the Kaiser Oakland Permanente Hospital where the nursing students would be working on staff as part of their training. As their month-long Christmas vacation approached, the students were settling into their new roles. Their transition from high school to nursing students had been made easier by Wangen's warm and supportive policies. This was about to change.

When the students returned from Christmas vacation with their families, they received a shock. Wangen was gone. There was no explanation. In her place was Dorothea Daniels, who had spent the past year as the Oakland hospital's assistant director of nursing. Dorothea Daniels was an excellent fit for Garfield's vision of a leader for the new school. The two quickly developed a mutually appreciative professional and personal relationship. There had been no question that Clare Wangen was competent and well-liked by the doctors, the hospital nurses and the students. However, she hadn't fit Sidney Garfield's vision of someone who could reshape nursing education by turning out graduates prepared to function effectively in a prepaid, nonprofit group practice setting with an emphasis on prevention while performing as an integrated part of the medical care team.

On the other hand, Daniels had a very impressive and perfectly suited résumé. She had trained at one of America's best nursing schools, Phillips Beth Israel School of Nursing at Mount Sinai Hospital in New York City. After graduation, she had enlisted in the Nursing Corps during World War I. Following the war, she'd worked as a night supervisor at Mount Sinai Hospital

while studying for a master's degree at Columbia University; she later earned a doctorate in education at New York University.

Daniels also had an outstanding background in nursing school administration. From 1936 to 1945, she had been director of her alma mater. She was passionate about her work.

DANIELS' VISION OF THE MODEL NURSE

While director at Phillips, she developed a vision of a well-trained, well-rounded nurse. She'd set high professional standards in both education and deportment. She made it clear that physical fitness also was required of a good nurse. According to the Phillips school's historians, "Daniels insisted on student nurses who looked healthy and fit, believing that if students were overweight, they could not work hard and take care of patients."[17]

This concept of "self-care" for nurses was precociously forward thinking.

In a paper published in the November 1940 American Journal of Nursing, "What Ninety Girls Like to Do in Their Spare Time," Daniels described why it was essential for students to find and participate in activities outside of school. She

This concept of "self-care" for nurses was precociously forward thinking.

was an early adopter of what is now termed "work-life balance," and thought if good nurses spent all their energy on patient care without setting aside time for recreation, family, sports or other hobbies, it was a sure path to burnout.[18] She had recognized the value of self-care for nurses decades before the idea became recognized as an antidote to burnout or "compassion fatigue."

Daniels also incorporated etiquette and social manners into students' nursing education and arranged for students to attend their first concerts or plays to introduce them to cultural experiences. This was a conviction Daniels continued with the new Permanente School of Nursing.

She had one other important conviction, one that must have resonated particularly well with Garfield. She thought it was a vital part of a nurse's job to educate patients so they could participate in their own health care. For Garfield, this was an important aspect of his new model of health care, and a natural outgrowth of prepaid group practice medicine. As Garfield often said, it was what made Kaiser Permanente a true heath plan, not one of the "sick plans" operated by indemnity insurance companies, doctors and hospitals that relied on patient illness for fee-for-service income. Years later, the Kaiser Permanente motto would sum this attitude up in a single word: "Thrive."

James Vohs, who served as president/CEO of the Kaiser Health Plan during a 50-year career with Kaiser, had worked closely with both Daniels and Garfield. He remembered Garfield saying that he didn't hire Daniels, that "Dorothea hired us."[19]

Pediatrician John Smillie, a Permanente pioneer and author of "Can Physicians Manage the Quality and Costs of Health Care?: The Story of The Permanente Medical Group," also worked closely with Daniels. He described her as being "… a crackerjack administrator: a trained nurse with a highly informed sense of medical responsibility, and a no nonsense, sometimes stern matriarch ruling physicians, nurses, and staff with total authority. Daniels's style [was] charismatic but highly individual."[20]

For students who had grown accustomed to the warmth and supportiveness of Wangen, Dorothea Daniels was an abrupt change. At age 53, with more than three decades of experience behind her, the new director took over her position with definite ideas of how a nursing school should be run.

The students soon nicknamed her the "Iron Nurse." Her carriage was ramrod straight, possibly a result of her time in the military. Her uniform was spotless, and starched with never a wrinkle, perhaps because she rarely sat down until the end of the day. She seemed to be in perpetual motion. Her immaculate uniform was topped off by a small upright organdy cap with black trim that identified her as a graduate of the Phillips Beth Israel School of Nursing.

Since it was traditional for each school of nursing to have a distinct uniform cap, Daniels designed a cap for the new school of nursing. The shape of the design of the cap was inspired by the Kaiser Industry logo. Later the School of Nursing adapted a version of the logo as its own. The cap had an embroidered "PH" for Permanente Hospital. The cap remained basically unaltered throughout the school years except for a change in 1953, when the school name was changed from "Permanente" to "Kaiser." In recognition of the name change, the "PH" became "K."

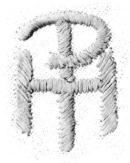

STUDENT LIFE

Janice Price Klein, Class of '63, later described nursing school life: "Entering KFSN can best be described as a cross between entering a finishing school, a nunnery, and joining the military. Just like the military there were many rules. Our schedules were not our own. We were told when to study, when lights went out, and what time to be

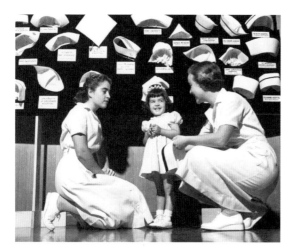

(Left) Child learns that each school of nursing has its own distinctive cap.

(Above) Embroidery on nurse's cap indicating she'd trained at the Permanente Hospital.

(Opposite) Study time in dorm room.

on duty, when we could accept phone calls or be off campus. We wore uniforms and were required to pass muster from our fingernails to our polished shoes. Our rooms had to pass inspection too, with beds neatly made each morning. The next three years were planned for us in terms of where we would rotate to and what few vacation days we had. Most of us were 17 or 18 years old, fresh out of high school, and would essentially grow up together during the next three years. Our house mothers did their best to truly watch over us, checking us in from dates, checking our rooms at night to make sure we were safe and sound. They were surrogate parents for the flock, good at listening, encouraging and hugging when words failed."[21]

By 10 o'clock when the front door was locked, students had to be in their rooms with the lights out. Later each night, Mrs. Irving, one of the early housemothers, would make her rounds with a flashlight. Using the old hotel's master key, she would check each room to make sure the students were there. While some students may have resented the intrusions and supervision, often comparing dormitory life to being in a convent, most remember these rules as providing a sense of being valued and safe.

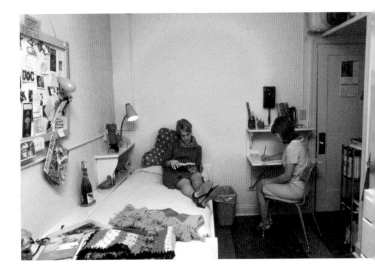

The students appreciated that the building had been designed as a hotel. Each room had a bathroom, rather than the usual dormitory arrangement of a large shared bathroom at the end of the hall.

Most rooms were doubles, not fancy but more than adequate. Even the new beds had a history of their own. They were war surplus originally purchased by the Kaiser shipyards to go to sea in Liberty and Victory ships, now repurposed for the landlocked student nurses.

Students stored their clothing in the built-in closet or in drawers beneath the beds. By the door was a small wall-hanging desk. Above it on the wall was a telephone that connected to the school switchboard on the first floor, another remnant of the building's original life as a hotel. Students could make only local calls on their room phones, and they were asked to keep them down to no more than 10 minutes. The most desirable rooms were on the ends of the corridors on each floor. These were roughly twice the size of the double rooms, but were assigned three students.

Ethel O'Donnell Morgan, class of '53B, explained how roommates were selected: "The director of nurses would not permit you to room with someone you knew. They took students from the end of the alphabet and put them with girls from the front of the alphabet. I wound up with Marilyn Anderson. I was Ethel O'Donnell. Then, after you had been there a year, you could change roommates if you wanted. I was angry that they did this because I didn't know Marilyn and I didn't want to room with her but then, at the end of the year, I didn't want to change and she didn't either. We're still friends today."[22]

Roommate selections for minority students were done differently. They were assigned to room together to ease their transitions into this new environment. In an interview many years later, Grace Oshita Miyamoto, class of '58, described her experience when she and Gladys Kashiwamura Jackson, another Japanese American student also from Lahaina, Hawaii, arrived in Oakland for their first year. They were not assigned according to the alphabet system but, like the others, they could not room with friends that first year.

"There were two other Japanese girls who were from Auburn. I ended up with one of the Auburn girls and Gladys ended up with the other. There were also two black girls in my class. One was Juliette Whitfield Powell, class of '58, and the other was Bettie Miller Williams. They ended up as roommates. During that time, I think they wanted to keep the different ethnicities together."

It is notable especially for this time in history, that in extensive interviews done for this book, no student or faculty member reported any instances or feelings of racial prejudice during their years at the nursing school, nor was there any sign of it in the school archives. Students of color reported this was the only nursing school in the area that made them feel welcome — there was no discrimination in enrolling students.

An active renunciation of discrimination and encouragement of diversity in its student body

*An active renunciation
of discrimination and
encouragement of diversity
in its student body were
clear examples of innovative,
courageous leadership and a
culture of inclusion in the face
of societal pressures that didn't
support these views. They were
to become powerful legacies
of Kaiser Permanente and
the Kaiser Foundation
School of Nursing.*

were clear examples of innovative, courageous leadership and a culture of inclusion in the face of societal pressures that didn't support these views. They were to become powerful legacies of Kaiser Permanente and the Kaiser Foundation School of Nursing.

Before enrolling in the nursing school, Naomi Eiko Tanikawa, class of '54A, experienced another

form of discrimination, and it actually led her to Kaiser. Since childhood, Tanakawa had wanted to be a lawyer. "I remember when I was a senior in high school down here in Long Beach, there was a student nurse that came with a cape and a cap. She was in the first class. She talked about being a nurse. I thought, oh, no. I wanted to be a lawyer."

Tanikawa had applied to the University of California's law school, (then known as) Boalt Hall, and had been admitted. "After I had paid my tuition and I'd paid for my room, I went over to Boalt Hall to be interviewed by a dean. You have to remember that this was right after World War II, and those of us who were Japanese were not rich. The dean didn't realize that Naomi was a female name; he probably thought it was a Japanese first name. In essence, what he said to me after a long conversation was, 'I cannot waste the state's money educating you because you are going to get married and have babies.'

"So instead of taking the bus down to downtown Oakland, I started walking. I walked down Broadway and there was this Kaiser Hospital and I remembered the student nurse that had come to the high school. Since I had all my transcripts and documents with me, I walked in. By

(Clockwise from left)
Sunbathing on dormitory roof.

School library was stocked with excellent nursing journals and textbooks.

The library was a comfortable place for research and study.

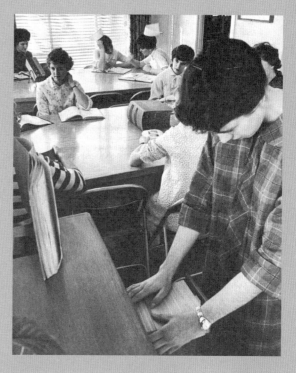

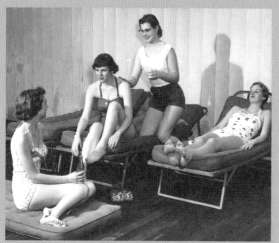

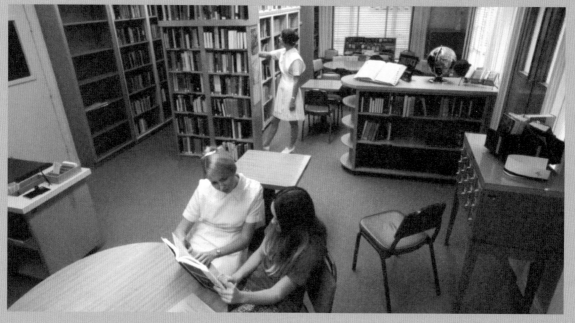

that time, I was halfway down to the Greyhound depot. I walked in and I think I was interviewed by Miss Gammell. She was the assistant director of nursing. She said 'You're too late for the next class. We'll take you for the one after that, which starts in January.'"[23]

One way the school tried to help students adjust to their new life was through a Big Sisters mentorship arrangement. As each new class arrived at the school, first-year students were assigned a Big Sister from the previous class to help her get oriented and make the transition between high school life and a professional medical education.

In addition to the student rooms, the school building contained a library well-stocked with medical books and current professional journals, thanks to the Kaisers' ongoing support.

The school building had no dining room because the students ate all their meals at the hospital. However, there was a kitchenette in the dormitory that had been squeezed into what had been the attic above the sixth floor, and a larger, better-stocked one in the basement.

Recognizing that these were active young women, the school supplied butter, peanut butter, milk, eggs and similar food. There was a refrigerator, stove and oven students could use to make something more ambitious than snacks, but they had to pay for the ingredients.

Student social life revolved around the dormitory. The students socialized and studied on the building's rooftop sundeck, and there was a comfortable common room on the second floor. The students could bring their dates there, but male guests were never allowed in the upstairs rooms. Often, several couples would be sitting in the common room listening to music and chatting. After repeated visits, the "gentlemen callers" would get to know each other, too, and friendships developed among the young men.

Students did not have a great deal of free time to spend with classmates, but all were facing the same challenges — they ate together, worked together and studied together and developed a sense of "we're all in this together." Lifetime friendships were formed. Instead of an atmosphere of competition, students supported each other. Francine Weir Ammerman described what that was like: "There was a lot of study time when we would go from one room to another to study … as a group, to throw questions at one another. We'd spend a lot of time in our classmates' rooms going over material to make sure we knew it for the exams."[24]

Daniels, in accordance with her belief that relaxation time was an important aspect of student life, arranged for outings, including dances at local colleges. The school also belonged to an association of nursing schools in the Bay Area that held an annual dance at the Claremont Hotel, one of the loveliest hotels in northern California, and where Henry Kaiser often entertained guests and conducted business meetings.

DOROTHEA DANIELS' INFLUENCE ON STUDENT EDUCATION AND COMPORTMENT

Dorothea Daniels appeared aloof to students, reserving her warmth for her dog, a tiny Pekingese who spent his "workdays" nested in the bottom drawer of her desk. The dog, named Fluffy, held special privileges and it wasn't uncommon for Daniels to ask students and even staff nurses to take him outside for walks and rest breaks.

It was particularly easy for her to keep an eye on the students because she was living with them. She shared a suite of rooms on the second floor of the residence with her assistant, Gladys Gammell, who had accompanied her from New York.

Students faced daily inspections of their fingernails, uniforms, shoes and caps, and they were all weighed regularly. Perfume was forbidden, as was all nail polish, even clear polish. Any infractions could lead to reprimands or a student being "grounded" for a time. And of course, marriage was grounds for immediate dismissal.

Students were given lessons in deportment, standing and sitting properly, and even learning to walk with books balanced on their heads.

Ethel O'Donnell Morgan, class of '53B, remembered how difficult it could be to please the school's director: "I was walking in the hall one day and Miss Daniels said, 'Miss O'Donnell, your hair is entirely too long. It is not allowed to touch your collar.' We had mandarin collars. 'Do something with your hair.' So, the next day I wore it up in a chignon. When Miss Daniels saw me she said, 'Miss O'Donnell that is a boudoir hairdo. Do not come to work looking like that.'"

This presented O'Donnell with a bit of a problem.

"I had no money for a hairdresser so one of my classmates chopped off my hair pretty short. When Miss Daniels saw it she asked, 'What did you do, run into a lawn mower? Your hair is entirely too short!'"[25]

Francine Weir Ammerman revealed more about Daniels when she recalled that her hobby was flying. "On weekends, that's what she did to relax. She had an airplane and she went flying. She added, "She wore a little gold ID bracelet — and nail polish which we were forbidden to do. We couldn't wear nail polish, no jewelry of any kind."[26]

Clair O'Sullivan Lisker, a member of the second class to be admitted to the school, remembered Daniels like this: "She wasn't a nurturing individual. She was stern in the view of the students." The awe in which she was regarded by the students almost had serious and lasting consequences for Lisker. "She didn't tolerate illness very readily. I can remember not feeling well for quite a while, just feeling terribly tired but not having a symptom that I could put my finger on. I woke up one day and I remember thinking, 'Oh, my, my eyeballs are yellow.' I had hepatitis. I had been complaining for at least two weeks that I wasn't feeling well. It wasn't until I became so jaundiced that I could see Director Daniels and tell her I was ill. Then I ended up in a hospital bed for six weeks and off duty for about three months."[27]

Daniels occasionally showed a more thoughtful, if not a tender side. She encouraged her best students to earn a bachelor's degree in addition to their RN diploma, believing that a well-rounded education would ensure a promising future. Lisker was one of those students. Daniels told her she wanted her to take the additional classes at College of the Holy Names so she could earn a bachelor's degree after obtaining her RN. When

Lisker told her she couldn't afford tuition, Daniels replied, "Don't worry about that. I'll pay your fee and you can pay me back."[28] Lisker took the courses as directed but noticed there were only occasional deductions from her student stipend. Apparently, Dorothea Daniels had paid the bulk of the tuition out of her own pocket.

Francine Weir Ammerman had reason to feel heartfelt gratitude for what was a tender "Daniels Moment." She was a member of the senior class and only three months from graduation. She had been engaged to a member of the Marine Corps Reserve for several months. Because marriage while a student was grounds for immediate expulsion, she and Jerry had decided to keep their engagement a secret.

She didn't wear her engagement ring on her hand but pinned it secretly inside her uniform. Then in June 1950, the North Koreans invaded the South and Jerry received orders to prepare to move out. His Marine unit was heading for combat in Korea. Francine and Jerry wanted to get married before he left for no one knew how long.

When Daniels heard that Ammerman's young man had been ordered to Korea, she made an exception. With Daniels' blessing, the newlyweds had a short honeymoon before he went overseas. A year later, when Ammerman had graduated and was working in the Oakland hospital, word came back that Ammerman's husband had been seriously wounded, Daniels again showed her tender side by going out of her way to be a comfort to the distraught wife until her husband returned safely from Korea.[29]

CLINICAL EDUCATION: HANDS-ON TRAINING

Daniels' overall approach to the clinical education of nurses at Phillips and then at Permanente was quite standard for the times. Nursing students were used to supplement the hospital staff, learning by doing in a contemporary form of apprenticeship while helping to relieve the continuing shortage of nurses. Conforming to both the classroom and hospital schedules placed a great deal of strain on the students, who often had to work split shifts. Even if they worked the night shift, they still were expected to attend the next day's classes.

Clair O'Sullivan Lisker described how they learned: "We had classes, but basically we learned on the job. We had multiple patients we were responsible for. We were staffing a hospital on the day shift, the evening shift and the night shift. On the night shift we'd have a wing of patients. It was horrendous, the responsibility. No wonder we grew up so quickly."[30]

She described her responsibilities as a student. "An average assignment duty in the morning would be probably six to eight patients for total care: bathing, ambulating, treatments, you name it — and then going to class in between. We'd have split shifts, but we'd come back after class to finish what we had to do or we'd have class after our shift."[31]

For their first days on the wards they were assigned to carry out the simple duties nurse's aides often performed. Even these simple tasks could turn out to be both memorable as well as unexpected, teaching them important lessons. Lesley Meriwether, class of '63, remembered her first day on the ward: "... we were only supposed to bring the trays to our patients. Very simple, minimum things. We each had two patients. My first patient was [a] thirty-eight-year-old man from

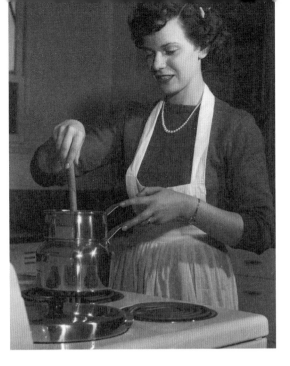

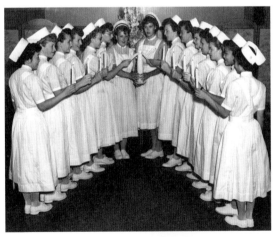

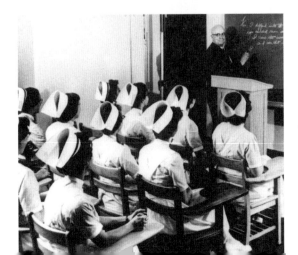

(Top to bottom) Francine Weir in Diet Kitchen Cooking Lab.

Capping Ceremony includes lighting the Nightingale Candle.

Henry J. Kaiser took a personal interest in the school.

Berkeley who'd had a heart attack — young. He was the father of two little girls and had a wife. He was sitting in the bed. I think it was the fourth day after his heart attack. There is a certain day when the recurrence is higher. ... I told him to relax and I would be back with his tray. I went to take the tray to my other patient first. When I went back to my first patient, he was lying on the floor. I immediately called for help. They couldn't save him. I didn't participate. I stepped back because I had no knowledge. I was literally the maid.

"It was pretty much overwhelming to me," Meriwether said. "I'd have a lot of deaths I was involved with and I learned how to deal with it. I grew stronger with all of them, but that first one was very traumatic for me."[32]

After a year of learning nursing fundamentals, students were ready for greater responsibilities. By the middle of their second year, they were integrated into the hospital staff, where they played an important role in hospital operations. They also began rotations to the various clinical specialties — three months in the operating room and obstetrics, plus six weeks in the diet kitchen and in Central Supply, sterilizing equipment. Carefully, deliberately, the supervisors

During MacLean's tenure, a massive reorganization and restructuring took place that disrupted the status quo of nursing education of that time. The school was decoupled from the hospital and students no longer were used to supplement hospital staffing.

and the school instructors increased students' responsibilities with increasing amounts of time with patients.

While there was no disputing the value of hands-on clinical experience, the strain it produced on students was not lost on Daniels' successor, Marguerite MacLean. During MacLean's tenure, a massive reorganization and restructuring took place that disrupted the status quo of nursing education of that time. The school was decoupled from the hospital and students no longer were used to supplement hospital staffing.

FACULTY

With her dual responsibilities as head nurse at the Permanente Hospital and administrator of the nursing school, Daniels had no time to teach, but some classes were led by Gladys Gammell, RN, her assistant. Gammell had graduated from Philadelphia General Hospital in 1928. She taught the nursing students *Materia medica* [pharmacology] and other subjects during her time at Permanente. However, most of the clinical instruction was done by the nursing supervisors of the various hospital departments, and by physicians.

One of Daniels' first goals was to enlarge the school's tiny faculty. There was a growing emphasis on specialization in nursing, so Daniels sought out nurses with advanced degrees, including those who, like herself, had earned doctorates. This gave her and the growing faculty greater control of the school's curriculum. According to Clair Lisker, "It was not a condition of employment but it was almost expected that you would go on and get a higher degree. Professionally, it was wise to do so if you wanted to go on in nursing."[33]

The school's education was strengthened by the fact these instructors' primary job was to teach. This contrasted with other schools of nursing, where students were taught by hospital supervisors, whose primary job was patient care.

It would take almost a decade to build up to a full nursing school faculty. One reason for the slow progress was Daniels' dual responsibilities that included directing nursing at the hospital. Although this made it easier for her to integrate students into the hospital, administration required much of her attention.

She hired nurses with advanced training to serve as role models for pursuing a nursing education beyond an RN diploma. Daniels herself was a model of professionalism. She demonstrated her conviction that nursing was an opportunity to connect deeply with patients, and that this connection was essential to patient care — what is now called creating a "healing environment."

Ammerman recalled from her student days that "the young women who were teaching us from the beginning were good role models; a little on the starchy side, but that's OK. We needed that. We were all pretty young and green. I think the instructors exemplified the attributes one would want in a nurse, and as time went on, we gravitated towards them."[34]

According to faculty member Bea Rudney, the new nursing instructors brought another change: "... they brought more of the humanitarianism, loving, caring role of nurses. The physicians were really scientifically oriented. ... I think nursing school faculty were very good role models. They were cooperative, they were approachable and they were current in their fields."[35]

Sharon Tolton Scolnick, class of '76, spoke for a lot of freshmen — reaching back to the earliest days of the school — when she recalled looking at students who already had been there for two years. She saw them carrying out their responsibilities and realized that "two years before, they were where you were now. We saw how self-assured they were. It was scary."[36]

Typically, patients welcomed the student nurses because of their unfeigned interest in them and because they had the feeling they were participating in the training of the next generation of nurses. Most of the physicians, too, enjoyed having the young women as students and treated them with consideration, perhaps like younger sisters. Some hospital personnel noted the nursing students often were treated better than the interns and residents.

In addition to academics, the school and the faculty were committed to protecting the health of their students, with an emphasis on self-care. But, no matter how careful the faculty was, there was a great deal of pressure involved in transforming high school students into highly competent nursing professionals in a little more than a thousand days. Bea Rudney, a graduate of the Cornell School of Nursing in New York City, joined the faculty in the late 1960s as health director for the student nurses.

"I cared very much for the students," Rudney said. "I really liked that age group. I kept them physically healthy and I tried very hard to keep them emotionally healthy because nursing is a profession [that] is very demanding. You are working with ill people, many of whom are dying. You need support for that. That was basically my job as health director."

Rudney often saw the results of this stress. "I took care of colds and cuts, things like that, but mostly it was moral support, reinforcement, showing them how they could cope. That was my main function."[37]

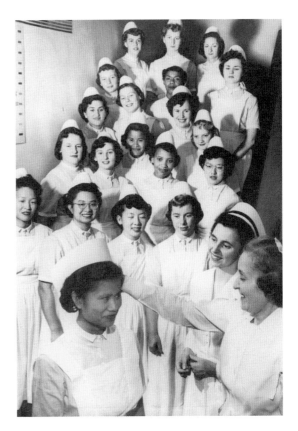

Capping ceremony 1952 with instructor Clair Lisker and director Dorothea Daniels: From the beginning, diversity of backgrounds was a hallmark of the school.

Marion Yeaw, who had a master's degree in nursing, joined the faculty in the early years of the school as the pediatric instructor. She remembered students she had helped over rough patches. Regarded by the students as one of the most demanding instructors, Yeaw had assigned her students to write a short, independent paper on some aspect of pediatrics that interested them. Each student could choose her own topic. One typically good student was having trouble with this assignment. She had done the research but was having difficulty writing the paper. Yeaw recalled the incident with obvious satisfaction.

Nightingale Pledge

"I solemnly pledge myself before God, and in the presence of this assembly, to pass my life in purity and to practice my profession faithfully. I will abstain from whatever is deleterious and mischievous and will not take or knowingly administer any harmful drug. I will do all in my power to maintain and elevate the standard of my profession and will hold in confidence all personal matters committed to my keeping and all family affairs coming to my knowledge in the practice of my calling. With loyalty will I endeavor to aid the physician in his work and devote myself to the welfare of those committed to my care."

"I sat down and showed her an outline. 'State your problem, how you went about researching it, what you found out and your conclusions.'" Using this guide, the student was able to write up her research. Yeaw recalled, "Her grammar and punctuation weren't too hot. She showed me the rough draft and I corrected things for her ... because she had put so much work in it. She typed it up and got an A!" The result was very gratifying for them both.[38]

PINNING AND GRADUATION CEREMONIES

The students were reminded of the high traditions of their chosen profession by rituals that were landmarks in student life. The practice of "swearing in" a member of a guild or profession is a very old tradition that continues in some professional schools. The Permanente School of Nursing conducted swearing-in events six months into the school year at the capping ceremony. Held at a church, the ritual carried with it a kind of nonsectarian spirituality that at the time was an important part of the culture of nursing education. The students, until now labeled "probies," short for "probationers," had completed the initial stage of their education that was really an

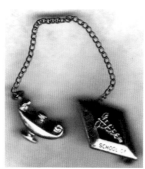

introduction to their profession. From that point on, they could consider they no longer were on probation and, as their knowledge and skills increased, they would be given increasing responsibility with patients.

To mark their new status, and in recognition of Florence Nightingale, the founder of modern nursing, the class recited the Nightingale Pledge, an adaptation of the 2,000-year-old Hippocratic Oath taken by physicians.

Forty students entered with the charter class of 1950 and about half of them made it to graduation. Most who dropped out left during the first few months, often because they realized nursing wasn't their calling. The realities of the training and the duties of the profession had come as an unwelcome surprise, and they had resigned. Over the coming years, that dropout rate would remain nearly constant, hovering at around 50 percent.

Those who chose to complete school found that the instructors often would go out of their way to help students who needed extra support or tutoring. The graduation rate likely would have been significantly lower if Rudney and other faculty members had not made the extra effort to encourage and support students through the academic and clinical obstacles they faced during three rigorous years.

Nurses from what would become the Kaiser Foundation School of Nursing earned a reputation for excellence based on their training, skills and leadership abilities. Their cap became a symbol they could be proud to wear. It followed that their performance as graduates enhanced the school's reputation wherever they went.

Innovations in nursing education and lasting legacies of the school of nursing were formed during the Daniels era. Many of these legacies shape the professional practice of nursing today: the values of preventive care, diversity and anti-discrimination, encouraging continuing education, a flourishing sense of community among students that built a culture of caring and teamwork, an emphasis on self-care, and life-balancing cultural and social development.

By 1953, after the graduation of four classes, it was clear that Dorothea Daniels had placed her individual stamp on nursing education at Kaiser Permanente — but this had come at a personal cost. "She regarded herself, and I think quite

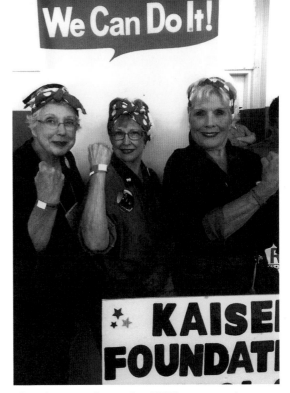

Three alumni proudly wear their KFSN caps on top of bandanas at a Rosie the Riveter "We Can Do It" event.

(Opposite) Worn on cap, this pin was awarded for successful completion of first year.

properly, as a peer of any of the doctors she was dealing with, said John Smillie, MD."[39] Her personality led to increasing resistance from the medical group. As a way of solving the growing problem, Sidney Garfield found a new challenge for her. He transferred her to the Kaiser Sunset Hospital in Los Angeles, where she became the first female administrator of a Kaiser Permanente Medical Center. Her departure would mark the beginning of the most significant changes in the history of the nursing school.

(Left) Dorothea Daniels, RN, MS,
EdD, Director 1948-1953.

(Right) Marguerite MacLean, RN
MSN, Director 1953-1958.

ERA of BREAKTHROUGHS

DIVERSITY, TEAMING WITH PHYSICIANS 3 AND INDEPENDENCE FROM HOSPITALS

The 1950s and the MacLean
Era of Innovative Education Breakthroughs

1953 — TRANSFORMATION AND REBIRTH FOR THE HEALTH PLAN AND SCHOOL OF NURSING The year 1953 was filled with great turmoil in what still was called the Permanente Health Plan. The medical care program had been under severe, sustained and vicious attack by a medical establishment that neither understood nor trusted the program, and that was threatened by the effect its continuing growth could have on the incomes of local physicians. The California Medical Society had become openly hostile toward the Health Plan, siding with the county medical societies against the prepaid group practice they unhesitatingly branded as unethical.

One reason for such animosity was that the Health Plan restricted members' choice of physicians to those in The Permanente Medical Group. They even called it "socialized medicine," which at the height of the McCarthy era was akin to insisting that anyone associated with the medical program was a Communist. Sidney Garfield's enemies even had managed to have his physician's license revoked on a technicality. Fairness and common sense prevailed and Garfield's license soon was restored, but whatever the motivations, at the heart of these attacks was the charge that the Kaiser organization was providing poor-quality medical care. This was despite the fact that measured by any unbiased yardstick, the truth decidedly was different. Both Garfield and Henry Kaiser remained targets of the fee-for-service physicians in an ongoing campaign to cripple or destroy the Health Plan.

Garfield's strategy for dealing with critics was straightforward. He invited critics to take a close-up look at their operation. He opened up the hospitals and their records to their inspection. The local medical societies took him up on the offer. Dr. Cecil Cutting, the first medical director of The Permanente Medical Group, described what happened: "They sent committees several times to look us over, but one thing they could never find was poor quality."[1]

Henry Kaiser also was subject to the medical establishment's attacks. In the early '50s, the Kaiser program still was known as the Permanente Health Plan, harkening back to its birth in Henry Kaiser's World War II Permanente shipyards. In 1953, in recognition of his contributions to the Health Plan, the Permanente Health Plan became the Kaiser Health Plan. However, another one of the persistent charges being made against Permanente was that it was controlled by Henry Kaiser, who profited from its services. If that had been true, it certainly would have been unethical. One of the canons of medical ethics was that physicians could only be employed by other physicians to avoid even the appearance that the treatment of patients was being directed by laymen. The physicians' group was asked whether it also would like to change its

Permanente name to Kaiser. For the physicians it was an easy choice. To make it crystal clear they were independent of Henry Kaiser and any other lay-person's control, the physicians turned down the Kaiser name. Ever since, they have remained The Permanente Medical Group,[2] a continuing reminder of their independence and integrity.

The same year that the Permanente Health Plan became the Kaiser Health Plan, there was another Permanente-to-Kaiser name change. When the Permanente School of Nursing became the Kaiser Foundation School of Nursing (KFSN), in 1953, it was far more than just a name change. Until this time, like most diploma nursing schools, the Permanente School of Nursing had operated as an extension of an associated hospital — in this case, Permanente in Oakland, California. Following the school's name change to Kaiser Foundation School of Nursing, the school operated as a part of the nonprofit Kaiser Foundation rather than as an extension of the hospital. This soon would have far-reaching implications for the philosophy and curriculum of the nursing school, legitimately staking its claim and position as a national leader in nursing education, and building a standard and legacy for nursing schools in the decades that followed.

Hospital-based, or apprentice models of nursing education were prevalent across the United States at this time, while degree programs were less common and more costly. While running a nursing school independently of a hospital was highly unusual at that time, it was not a new idea. In fact, Florence Nightingale had proposed that nursing schools be financially independent of any service institutions with which they are affiliated.[3]

From 1948, soon after the school's founding, until 1953, the school had thrived under the leadership of Dorothea Daniels. She had established high standards and the curriculum continually was refined and improved. The students knew and appreciated the quality of the education they were receiving. That appreciation and the established traditions that became a part of the school culture ensured a student body loyal to both the school and to each other.

Year after year the entering classes grew larger. As each class completed its three years, graduates found positions in the Oakland, California hospital and in other Kaiser and non-Kaiser facilities. Wherever they went, their training and professionalism reflected extremely well on their alma mater.

However, during this time, a problem became increasingly evident. At its center was Dorothea Daniels, who not only set high standards for students and faculty at the nursing school, but demanded the same sort of professionalism from the hospital nursing staff and physicians. Daniels did not hesitate to let physicians know when they were not living up to her standards. Resentment about the way she treated them began to build among the medical staff, until it interfered with her effectiveness in the hospital and to some degree in the school.

That was why, in that already eventful year of 1953, Garfield found himself facing a difficult decision. It was becoming clear that his friend, a woman he respected for her administrative and leadership skills, was going to have to go. Daniels seems to have understood Garfield's dilemma and helped identify who should succeed her. Jointly, they selected Marguerite MacLean to head the nursing school.

As a part of the reorganization, the governance of the school was separated from the hospital. Grace Gurney took over as director of nursing at the hospital so MacLean could put all of her energies into running KFSN.

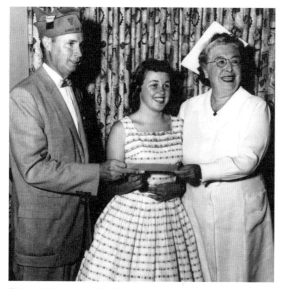

*Director Marguerite MacLean giving
a scholarship to a student nurse.*

MacLean, who had received her nursing education from the University of California, San Francisco, already had demonstrated her academic and management abilities as the successful director of Highland Hospital and Nursing School, also in Oakland, California. She was available because the board at Highland Hospital had been unwilling to give her the salary increase she thought she had earned and deserved. Permanente offered her an alternative.

In addition to her professional qualifications, there were other not-so-obvious political reasons she was an excellent choice. By 1953, the Kaiser Health Plan had been growing rapidly, and it now was more of a competitive economic force potentially threatening the income of the local doctors. Its success was a major reason it remained under sustained attack by the fee-for-service physicians. Garfield also knew MacLean could help with his critics. She had a firm grasp on the realities of medical politics in California. Her brother, H. Gordon MacLean, was a major figure in that arena. In 1950, he had been elected unanimously to the post of president of the California Medical Association.[4]

As for Dorothea Daniels, Garfield expressed his continuing confidence in her by appointing her administrator of the new Kaiser Hospital in Los Angeles—a move that made her the first woman to hold such a position in the Kaiser system. Following her success there, she was assigned to the same position at the Kaiser Hospital in San Francisco, to solve its persistent administrative problems.

MAKE US RESPECTABLE

It was during this same period that Garfield and Kaiser, reacting to the attacks by fee-for-service medicine, had hired Clifford Keene, MD to take over running the Health Plan, giving him the deceptively simple instruction, "make us respectable." Keene interpreted this to mean, "Do whatever you need to do to earn the respect, even if it is grudging, of the medical community in general." His new responsibilities, he understood, included the nursing school.

The vagueness of "make us respectable" left Keene wondering where to begin. Soon after his arrival in Oakland, California, he found himself in a meeting with Henry Kaiser's older son, Edgar. Henry Kaiser also was there but was preoccupied. His thoughts were miles away. He was not participating in the conversation, at least not until Keene mentioned he had some ideas for changes in the school of nursing that would result in cost savings. Suddenly the industrialist was alert. He sat up abruptly. Succinctly and powerfully, Kaiser told Keene to keep his hands off the nursing school. This wholehearted support from Henry Kaiser was indicative of the financial and administrative independence now available to the school. Although Keene's ideas for the nursing school initially were not welcomed by Kaiser, Keene ultimately developed a strong appreciation for Marguerite MacLean and her impact on the quality of the education offered by the school of nursing.[5]

RESTRUCTURING THE SCHOOL

The change of administration from Daniels to MacLean marked the beginning of major changes in the evolution of what now would be known as the Kaiser Foundation School of Nursing. The new name was a clear signal that the school no longer was a part of the Health Plan, nor a subsidiary of the hospital. It was now a freestanding educational institution, no longer responsible to the hospital administration but to the Kaiser Foundation that provided the school with both a governing board and financial backing. That same year, the school received accreditation from the National League for Nursing, fulfilling Garfield's objective of having "an accredited school of nursing."

Many members of the board of trustees were executives in Kaiser Industries, giving the school access to the formidable business skills of that corporation's top executives. Furthermore, the design of the school's cap, which reflected the company logo, was a steady reminder of the school's connection to the Kaiser organization.

Another indication of the importance and respect the school now enjoyed was that MacLean reported directly to Keene, who in turn reported directly to Kaiser. With the enthusiastic encouragement of Henry Kaiser and the financial resources of the Kaiser Foundation to draw upon, MacLean was able to hire additional faculty members with advanced degrees and specialized training in OB/GYN, med-surg and orthopedics. The school soon had a panel of dedicated faculty members whose primary goal was education, not patient care.

New faculty members brought various approaches to their specialties. Students were taught how to care for hospitalized patients and the importance of planning for their home care after release. They learned to instruct family members on post-discharge home care, and how to design

treatment plans that even included what services the patient might need if he or she had to return to the hospital. This was not a state nursing board requirement, but the faculty thought it emphasized the value of continuity of patient care and included it as part of the school's curriculum.

This mindset of setting a bar above and beyond the regulatory requirements and expectations in the name of excellence in education and patient care explains how KFSN established so many legacies of innovation that inform, influence and remain relevant in nursing education.

Bea Rudney, one of the faculty members who oversaw home visits that were a part of the treatment

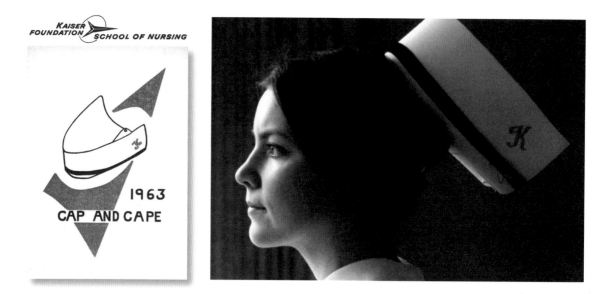

> *This mindset of setting a bar above and beyond the regulatory requirements and expectations in the name of excellence in education and patient care explains how KFSN established so many legacies of innovation that inform, influence and remain relevant in nursing education.*

plans said, "I would accompany the student to the home of a patient that they had cared for in the hospital. Yes, people with heart conditions, with lung conditions, to see how they were functioning at home, what kind of help they had and if they were carrying through on the discharge orders, things like that. That hadn't been done before."[6]

Perhaps the most important change during this time, and a radical innovation that put nursing education on a course that's standard practice today, was that the school stopped staffing the hospital with students.

Decoupling a school from a hospital so that the curriculum determined clinicals and hands-on learning (and not a hospital's staffing needs) was a significant, game-changing innovation in nursing education and a powerful legacy of the Kaiser Foundation School of Nursing. This shift directly led to increasing excellence in nursing education.

The school's expansion meant MacLean and her new faculty now had greater control over the curriculum. This allowed for a more organized and efficient use of both classroom and clinical time.

The school's primary goal was to produce nurses who could work in a prepaid integrated group practice with a focus on prevention and wellness, rather than in the fee-for-service environment far more common in postwar America. As Garfield had discovered in his desert hospital, an integrated system of health care where the insurance company, medical staff and hospital were all part of the same organization led inevitably to an emphasis on prevention. It was clear that the newly renamed Kaiser Foundation School of Nursing, under the direction of Marguerite MacLean (or Maggie as she was known to colleagues, and referred to by students, although not to her face), was not merely dedicated to turning out highly trained registered nurses, but also to providing the nursing profession with a corps of future leaders in clinical care, administration and research.

New faculty members were selected for their experience as well as their advanced educational accomplishments and degrees. They also served as role models to young women just starting out in nursing. An RN diploma might only be a beginning. They could go as far as they wished in their postgraduate education. In fact, the expectation was that graduates would become leaders whether they chose to dedicate their professional careers to clinical patient care or to move into administrative roles. The emphasis on the value of continuing education and the expectation that nursing students would assume leadership positions were both legacies of KFSN.

Janice Price Klein, class of '63, said: "Kaiser was just a starting point. You were to go on. You were to be the best you could be. You would need education the rest of your life to do that. You would need to educate others. You're going to be a leader. You were going to educate your staff. I don't think that there was anyone who graduated from Kaiser who didn't move into some influential role, including those who chose to remain at the

bedside — they were leaders as clinical nurses. We were groomed to be leaders. You were going to be among the movers and shakers."[7]

Of course, patient care still was central to student training, but the circumstances were very different than they had been before MacLean's arrival. Under careful faculty supervision, new students were introduced to working with patients starting with mastering routine nursing functions: taking blood pressures and temperatures, bed-making, toilet care and bed baths. Then, instead of staffing the hospital and caring for several patients at once, they were assigned to a single patient, gradually increasing their patient load and responsibilities as they became more competent in providing patient care.

Before 1953, it had been standard practice to assign students to care for several patients simultaneously. The emphasis necessarily had been on the "what" of nursing — what to do to care for the patient. Students had to learn about a disease, its progression, the particular patient's condition, the medications he or she was receiving, possible side effects and contraindications, and the danger signals to watch out for. Under the new model, starting with care of a single patient (and

"*Kaiser gave us a great education. I was really proud of my education. I learned how to be a good surgical scrub nurse. I learned a lot about all the different fields, OB and general nursing, because where I worked it was a very small hospital and we had to do all those things. I was kind of like a floating nurse.*"[8]

NANCY HORIE SUDA, CLASS OF '51A

"*I think we got a great education. We'd had outpatient as well as inpatient experience. We had a well-rounded education. I hadn't liked outpatient. I thought it was boring. I didn't want to do it but I'd had to. It was part of our education. Now I am glad I did.*"[9]

ETHEL O'DONNELL MORGAN, CLASS OF '53B

"*The young women who were teaching us from the beginning were good role models. I think the instructors exemplified the attributes one would want in a nurse, and as time went on we gravitated towards them.*"[10]

FRANCINE WEIR AMMERMAN, CLASS OF '50

Legacies: Key Elements of KFSN that Live On in Nursing Today

1. Autonomous school
2. Curriculum-driven clinicals
3. Diversity and inclusion
4. Zero tolerance for discrimination
5. Advanced education and academic partnerships
6. Lifelong learning and development
7. Interprofessional education
8. Clinical rotations went beyond the hospital
9. Care across the continuum
10. Critical thinking
11. Taught to be leaders and educators
12. Professional confidence and accountability
13. Qualified and prepared faculty
14. Integrated approach to create healing environments
15. Learned to be integral members of health care team
16. Cultural and social development
17. Self-care as a foundation for nursing
18. Flourishing sense of community and family
19. Taught to implement the Permanente way of practicing medicine
20. Innovation in education and health care

See list of legacies in the Appendix.

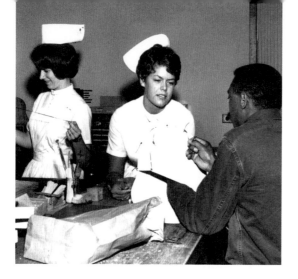

then later two), more of the students' time and effort could be spent on the "why" of treatment. Students were taught to listen carefully so they could see the patient as a whole person.

Physicians also were involved with teaching students the medical and pathophysiology aspects of an illness. The doctors often included students on rounds along with the interns and residents. Deloras Plake Jones, class of '63, remembers doctors inviting her to see patients and learn how physicians were assessing them, and showing her what she should look for in a patient.

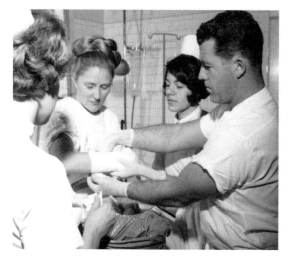

Incorporating Kaiser physicians and specialists in the classroom and in clinical settings was an interprofessional education model that developed collegial relationships between physicians and KFSN graduates, and it was a concept foundational to team-based care. It upended and disrupted the status quo of these relationships, all in the service of creating higher-quality education and clinical training.

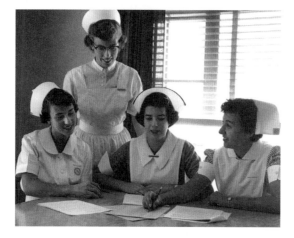

(Top to bottom) KFSN students on rotation – VA Hospital, Palo Alto, California.

TPMG physician teaching students how to set a cast for a broken arm.

KFSN students on outside rotations met students from other schools.

Matching patients to students was not random. The faculty made sure the students' clinical responsibilities were carefully synchronized with their classroom training. What they learned in the classroom would be applied immediately on the nursing floor, and what they saw in their patients gave increased depth and meaning to their classroom work. Helen Harrison Robinson, class of '65, described it this way: "We were always responsible for understanding the care that we gave. We weren't just taking orders. If we were given an order that we did not agree with, we had to be accountable, so we went through stacks of information."[11]

Having assumed some of the responsibility for patient care, the student had become a member of the patient care team. Robinson added, "You were part of a team of people. It's not just one person who holds all the knowledge. You have a lot of knowledge about what is going on with that patient." Learning to practice as a part of a team was an important element of a KFSN education, just as it was an important element in the prepaid group practice of the Health Plan.[12]

ROTATIONS

While clinical training necessarily was centered around the hospital in Oakland, California, there were some specialties the Oakland hospital was not equipped to support. The faculty thought it was necessary to affiliate with other medical institutions where students would have access to a wider variety of medical and, in the future, psychiatric conditions.

Incorporating Kaiser physicians and specialists in the classroom and in clinical settings was an interprofessional education model that developed collegial relationships between physicians and KFSN graduates, and it was a concept foundational to team-based care. It upended and disrupted the status quo of these relationships, all in the service of creating higher-quality education and clinical training.

Several times during their years at KFSN, students were assigned, usually in three-month blocks, to other medical facilities for specialized training in obstetrics and gynecology, psychiatry, contagious diseases and rehabilitation. Hospital affiliations for these specialties rotations were adapted to meet circumstances and the Kaiser Health Plan's need for specialized nursing. Students' psych rotation might be at the Stockton State Hospital or at the Veterans Hospital in Palo Alto, or later at the VA facility in Martinez.

For several years, the contagious disease affiliation was with the San Francisco County Hospital. Some hospital affiliations were at other Kaiser facilities, such as OB/GYN at what was then the brand-new Kaiser Hospital in San Francisco, or rehabilitation nursing at the Kaiser facilities in Vallejo or Santa Monica. There were even rotations in industrial medicine at the southern California Kaiser hospital at the Kaiser Steel Mill in Fontana, which provided the students with valuable clinical experience.

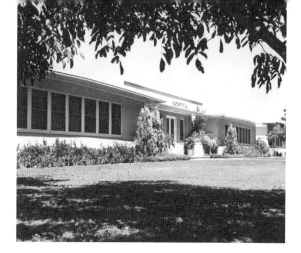

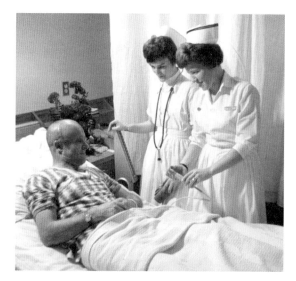

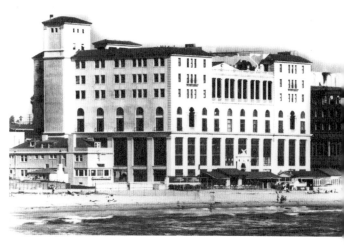

(Top to bottom) Fontana Hospital.

Instructor and student giving a patient discharge instructions.

Kaiser Permanente Rehabilitation Center on the Santa Monica beach.

Another important rotation for students was in the ambulatory care clinics. The clinics changed as the curriculum changed, so that outpatient rotations in OB, pediatrics, adult medicine and surgery occurred concurrently with those in the inpatient setting, giving the student the experience of care across the continuum and the opportunity to learn the value of the whole spectrum of care.

As part of his continuing support of the school, Henry Kaiser provided cars for the students' commute, including Kaiser-manufactured vehicles. Students commuted daily from Oakland in a carpool to the various sites and returned to the dormitory and their classmates each night.

"When we went out to other hospitals, to our affiliations, they would say (in a sneering tone) 'You go to Kaiser? That's socialized medicine. What could you be learning there?' Then, after they had worked with us a while, we became the ones they wanted to work with, because we knew what we were doing." [13]

PHYLLIS PLANT MORONEY, CLASS OF '57A

During their rotations at outside medical institutions, Kaiser students met young women and men from other nursing schools and had the opportunity to measure themselves and their training against the other students' experience.

Henry and Bess Kaiser had a special interest in rehabilitation medicine. In 1945, when their son Henry Jr. was diagnosed with multiple sclerosis, the Kaisers had searched nationwide for someone who could help him. In searching for their son's effective treatment, Garfield found Dr. Herman Kabat in Washington, D.C. Kabat had developed what he called proprioceptive neuromuscular facilitation, a treatment that had offered some immediate relief to the young Kaiser. Heartened by this, Henry and Bess brought Kabat to Vallejo where they established the Kabat-Kaiser Institute, now KFRC, the Kaiser Foundation Rehabilitation Center. Shortly after that, Kabat-Kaiser expanded to the Santa Monica facility. Both developed excellent reputations for the innovative care offered to people suffering from multiple sclerosis, strokes and spinal cord injuries. Today, students come from all over the world to attend KFRC's postgraduate training in Kabat's technique, philosophy and patient handling skills.

So easy to see...

Kaiser's the car !

1951 Kaiser DeLuxe 4-Door Sedan. One of 6 body styles, 12 models. Hydra-Matic drive available in all models at extra cost.

1951 Kaiser ...the only car with Anatomic Design !

1951 Kaiser sedan wins world's highest honor Grand Prix d'Honneur Cannes, France

So pleasing to the eye...so easy to see *out* of! The new 1951 Kaiser gives more windshield and window area than any other passenger car... 1096 square inches in the windshield *alone*! The slim, slant-back corner posts eliminate "blind spots"...give you *Control-Tower Vision*...one of the many features of Kaiser's Anatomic Design that increase your safety, comfort, convenience!

Winner of the Grand Prize of Honor at Cannes, France, the 1951 Kaiser offers *everything* you've ever desired in a fine motor car. And everything is designed for the years ahead! Feature for feature, the 1951 Kaiser is the newest thing on wheels—in styling...engineering ...and comfort! See it at your Kaiser-Frazer dealer's now!

© 1951 KAISER-FRAZER SALES CORPORATION, WILLOW RUN, MICHIGAN

Built to Better the Best on the Road!

In the early '50s, Kaiser was operating the two rehabilitation centers, Vallejo and Santa Monica, and student rotations were split between the two facilities. Students who went to Santa Monica were housed on an attractive, palm-lined beachfront in a hospital that not long before had been a luxurious hotel. In contrast, students assigned to Vallejo spent their three-month rehab rotation in a daily 40-mile commute from Oakland. Rotation assignments remained split between Vallejo and Santa Monica until Vallejo expanded enough to have adequate patients, personnel and facilities to train all the nursing school students. This had the added advantage of allowing students to be "closer to home." Instead of being away from the school during their rotation, students remained on campus, living in the dormitory.

Grace Oshita Miyamoto, class of '58, was one of four students in her class whose rehab rotation assignment was the luxurious Kaiser facility on the Santa Monica beachfront.[14] The four were given two corner rooms on the top floor of the resort hotel turned hospital. The other rooms on their floor were reserved for patients who'd been attracted by Kabat-Kaiser's worldwide reputation. Although these patients needed extensive physical therapy and perhaps crutches or even a wheelchair to get about, they were able to care for themselves and did not need the full services available in the wards below.

At Santa Monica, caring for the spirits of the patients was as much a priority as caring for their bodies. Miyamoto recalled a fall day at Santa Monica when one of her classmates suggested a special Halloween celebration — to take the pediatric patients trick or treating. Her classmates were excited by the idea; using what they could scavenge from around the hospital, they created costumes and masks.[15]

The children, many with serious disabilities, were thrilled with this adventure. "We took them upstairs to the top floor," Miyamoto recalled. "We had told the people up there that we were going to be taking the kids trick or treating and we would be knocking on their doors. When I look back at that I think, 'Wasn't that wonderful for those kids who were hospitalized!!'"[16]

The KFSN students had created a win-win-win situation. The children were delighted with the idea, the adult patients on the top floor enjoyed seeing the youngsters' pleasure, and the student nurses had a wonderful time bringing joy to the young patients and the other residents of the top floor. Miyamoto smiled as she remembered that Halloween: "The little ones were just so happy! That was so rewarding when I look back at that."[17]

Miyamoto recalled that she and her classmates thought about their patients all the time while assigned to the Santa Monica facility, even during their time off. During her rotation in 1957, the students got permission to take a station wagon belonging to the institute on the 42-mile trip from Santa Monica to the recently opened Disneyland. They decided to share their outing. They invited a post-polio patient from Iowa living at the institute who didn't have many opportunities to get away from the hospital, and who only could travel with the aid of a helper. Many decades later, the memory of the pleasure they gave to this patient at "The Happiest Place on Earth" brought another smile to Miyamoto's face. This sort of caring was fostered by the school, and that was a legacy she and her classmates carried with them throughout their careers.[18]

As Health Plan membership continued to grow, Kaiser's hospital facilities expanded and diversified, rendering many of the outside affiliations unnecessary. Training experiences now were

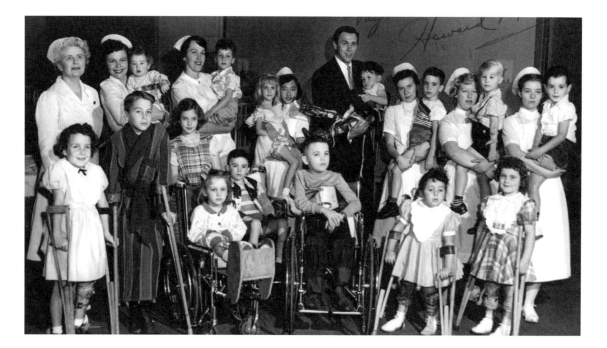

available closer to the school. Kaiser Oakland hospital became an increasingly busy place offering a wide variety of patients for students to care for and learn from. Rebecca Schoenthal Calloway, class of '61, summed this up: "Because Kaiser in Oakland had such a conglomeration of different patients, you saw everything from the loneliest man you've ever seen dying of cancer to a Berkeley professor. I remember [being] a silly little nursing student and explaining to the professor that his intravenous solution was saline and what saline is. Later I found that he had won the Nobel Prize for Chemistry."[19]

OB-GYN ROTATION

The rotations in obstetrics and gynecology started at the Oakland hospital. When it became clear there were more OB/GYN learning opportunities available at the new Kaiser hospital in San Francisco, the rotation was moved there. Among the many innovations the student nurses were exposed to was a new version of rooming-in. It was nicknamed the "baby in a drawer." A new mother

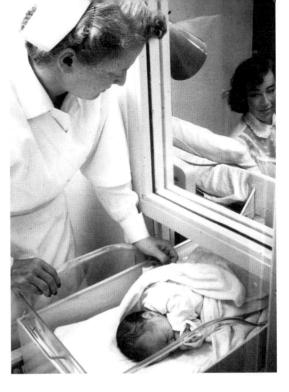

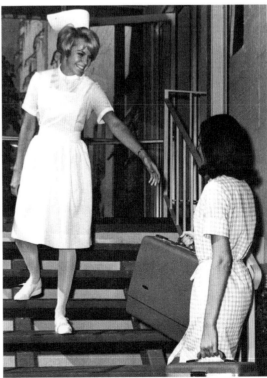

(Opposite) 50's movie star Howard Keel visiting students and patients at Kaiser Foundation Rehabilitation Institute in Santa Monica.

(Top to bottom) "Baby in a Drawer," an early and innovative form of rooming-in.

Her "Big Sister" greets arriving freshman.

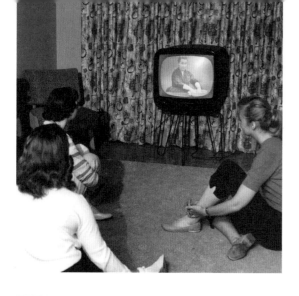

could keep her newborn with her as long as she wished, but when she was tired or wanted to rest, she could place the infant in a bassinet contained in a drawer beside the bed. A gentle push and the drawer slid through the wall into the nursery on the other side, where the charge nurse was notified immediately that the infant was there. A tug on the drawer, and the baby was back with its mother.

DORM LIFE

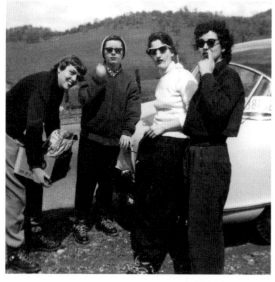

Life in the dormitory was an important part of KFSN nursing education. As soon as they arrived to begin their first year, the school administration helped new students feel welcome and at ease by assigning each incoming freshman a "Big Sister," a member of the previous class. Over the next two years, the Big Sister answered questions and generally was supportive. In addition to these assigned mentors, students formed lifelong friendships with their classmates. Many students were away from home for the first time. Living, studying, eating and working together created deep bonds of friendship. Lynn DeForest Robie, class of '57B, summed it up: "Living together 24 hours a day, you knew everybody. It was impossible not to. We were a part of each other's lives."[20]

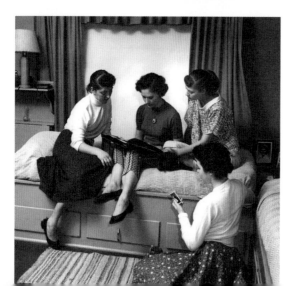

(Top to bottom) *Students relaxing in Common Room at Piedmont Hotel.*

Off on a holiday.

Studytime in dorm room.

The dormitory became a community. In the evenings in the dormitory, the young women had a chance to talk about their day, share experiences they'd had with instructors, patients, nurses and doctors, and discuss boyfriends, parent troubles and other personal issues. There was always a lot to talk about.

As you would expect from a group of high-spirited young women, "high jinks" or practical jokes were a part of dormitory life. Students returning from a weekend at home might find that the classmates who'd remained in the dormitory had short-sheeted their beds or placed strange objects beneath the covers. Some other tricks were in more questionable taste. One popular practical joke over the years was Saran Wrap stretched below a toilet seat. Other students found outlets for their high spirits and energy in such sports as races down the long upstairs corridors. Girls raced on their hands and knees as classmates standing along the improvised track cheered on their favorites.

Some classes put on an evening of skits to entertain themselves and invited guests, including family, faculty and medical staff. One skit had a group of students dressed elaborately as toys that climbed out of a toy box. Then, Katherine (Nelle) Neighbor

Alonzo, class of '71, dressed in a Western outfit as a cowboy, sang "They Call the Wind Mariah."[21]

Sometimes the girls added a bit of humor and gentle teasing of the faculty to their productions. One of the earlier classes performed a skit in which Daniels was portrayed as giving a steady stream of instructions and suggestions to a student representing Dr. Paul Fitzgibbon, one of the physician-leaders in Oakland, California, and a founder of The Permanente Medical Group. As the two crossed the stage on a set representing a hospital corridor, the audience could see that "Dr. Fitzgibbon" was mildly annoyed by "Miss

Born to Be a Nurse!

Nelle Neighbor is not only a KFSN graduate, she is the daughter of Wallace "Wally" Neighbor, MD, a founding member of the Permanente Medical Group who originally joined Sidney Garfield and Associates at Grand Coulee Dam where he met and married nurse Winifred Wetherill. Their daughter, Nelle, born in Oakland, became the first baby born in a Kaiser hospital.

Daniels'" persistence. When they reached the other side of the stage and a door clearly marked "Men's Room," the beleaguered physician escaped through it, saying, "Miss Daniels, there are some things a man has to do for himself."

Study hours began at 7 p.m., and the whole dormitory quieted down. The library was a popular study site, but most students chose to return to their rooms or gathered in small study groups to prepare for tests. They would fire potential test questions at each other in an atmosphere of cooperation rather than competition until they mastered the material.

After Bess Kaiser's death in April 1951, Henry remarried. His new wife was a nurse, Alyce (Ale) Chester, who had been an assistant to Garfield. The newlyweds had moved to Lafayette, a suburb of San Francisco, and in the years before they moved to Hawaii they would host a poolside party for the nursing school's senior class. Sometimes Henry Kaiser would join them in a game of volleyball, but it was understood that although he might serve the ball, it would be appreciated if it wasn't returned to him so he didn't have to get too involved in a spirited volley.[22]

STATE BOARD OF NURSING EXAMINATION

As the senior class prepared for the state boards, tension among students grew. There was a definite feeling that not only were their own futures at stake, but they were about to be representatives of the quality of a Kaiser Foundation School of Nursing education. MacLean assured them they didn't need to study too hard for the boards because if they hadn't learned the material already, it was too late to learn it. It's not clear whether this calmed many of the nervous seniors.

Faculty, too, was very interested in the results of the state nursing boards. At that time, board tests were divided by specialty. While the students received only pass or fail notices, the school received the students' actual grades in each specialty. Faculty members could see how each student fared in their fields, as could their colleagues and MacLean. The test results created an additional incentive for continuing improvements in teaching methods and curricula.

Over time, the results were heartening, trending steadily upward during MacLean's administration. KFSN students consistently scored among the top three California nursing schools.

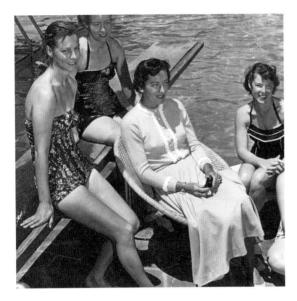

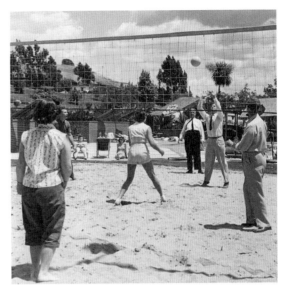

(Left to right) Ale Kaiser hostessing students
at Kaiser home, Lafayette, California.

Henry J. Kaiser (far side of net) joins pick-up
volleyball game with student guests.

Not only did the school take great pride in students' test results, so did the entire Kaiser organization. The August 1959 issue of the KP Reporter, "Published monthly for the Kaiser Foundation Medical Program," sported a headline: "STATE RATES KAISER NURSING SCHOOL HIGH." According to the article, while the California State Board of Nurse Examiners did not give out specific ranking details of each school's performance, the KFSN students in the class of 1958 had finished between first and fourth place among the 41 nursing schools in California, including the seven nursing schools affiliated with colleges. The school had been notified that their students had come in first in surgical nursing and near the top in medical, pediatric, obstetric and psychiatric nursing. The board added that these results were all the more impressive since, overall, California nursing schools performed substantially better than the national average on comparable tests. KFSN was proving itself to be among the best of the best.

The KP Reporter article went on to point out that the class of '58 was also the first to graduate after a curriculum change that replaced the study of nursing theory in their first year before starting their practice of medicine. Instead, the students went through a concentrated period of learning a foundation of basic nursing skills, and then quickly moved on to a program of classwork coordinated with appropriate patients who were being treated for the condition they were studying in the classroom. The implication was that continually upgrading the curriculum resulted in the outstanding test performance. This sort of coordination of class and clinical had proven so successful that it was intensified and shifted to begin earlier.

Juliette Whitfield Powell, class of '58, was a member of the class lauded in the KP Reporter article. She and her classmate, Christina Busey Irvin, had received the highest scores in the state. "Almost from Day One," Powell said, "we'd had a set number of hours in the hospital doing blood pressures, temperatures, basic nursing care with an instructor." She compared her experience at KFSN with that of students at the nearby Highland Hospital nursing school, as well as most other nursing schools at the time. "That was different than at Highland. We were never used in place of an RN," she said. "We had to make it to class. That's why we did so well on state boards — because we could not miss our classes where at Highland, you could not go to class unless you had finished your work because they did use the students as personnel. Kaiser never did that. We were never used as personnel, so we got a better book education. We were also well trained. One day after graduation, we could walk into a hospital and work."[23]

The high marks on state boards continued. In his history of The Permanente Medical Group, John Smillie, MD, wrote, "In 1967, for instance, graduates of the school placed first among 65 nursing schools including 4-year universities in three subjects: medical nursing, surgical nursing and pediatric nursing."[24]

RECRUITING STUDENTS

As the school's faculty expanded and training opportunities for the students grew, the school increased the size of its student body each year. Faculty and students became volunteer recruiters. They traveled to high schools in northern and central California and spoke to school nurses who in many cases also were the faculty advisers to nursing clubs. Recruiters made sure students understood the opportunities available at Kaiser. They also spoke to the students directly. Clair O'Sullivan Lisker, faculty member and a 1951 graduate, recalled how the recruiters concentrated on high school sophomores and juniors. She said of that time, "We tried to get them earlier so they could take the right classes, so they could come into the school. We didn't wait until they were seniors."[25]

The reasons a girl might choose a nursing education were many and varied. Many chose nursing because they had a passion for what it meant to be a nurse. Other girls were searching for an alternative to being a secretary or teacher, and some were anxious to get away from home. In those days, when all airline flights had a stewardess who was also an RN, some students saw a nursing education as a way to see the world. However, for most of them, no matter why they wanted to go to nursing school, the cost of a KFSN education was a major factor.

TUITION-FREE EDUCATION

A big advantage of the school's new status of being affiliated with the Kaiser Foundation was the generous financial support it provided. Because of that support, tuition, room, board, books and uniforms were free until 1957. Tuition was initiated that year, but because it still was subsidized by the Kaiser Foundation, it remained very low. Tuition for the three-year course in 1957 was $656, so the school still was within financial reach of young women of modest means who wanted a professional education.

Kaiser Foundation support also made it possible for the school to have a comprehensive professional library stocked with up-to-date textbooks, reference books and professional journals. To help students take full advantage of the facility, MacLean hired a professional librarian, who helped students with their research and scanned publishing lists for the best current professional publications to add to the school's collection and keep it current.

There was also a lighter side to the library. The wives of the physicians were enthusiastic supporters of the students and instructors at the school. They went through their personal book collections and donated books for students' recreational reading. As a result, mixed in with the most current medical and nursing journals on the library shelves was a generous selection of mysteries, biographies and romance novels.

Even though tuition was very low, it still was comprehensive and included their meals, dormitory housing, medical care and uniforms as well as

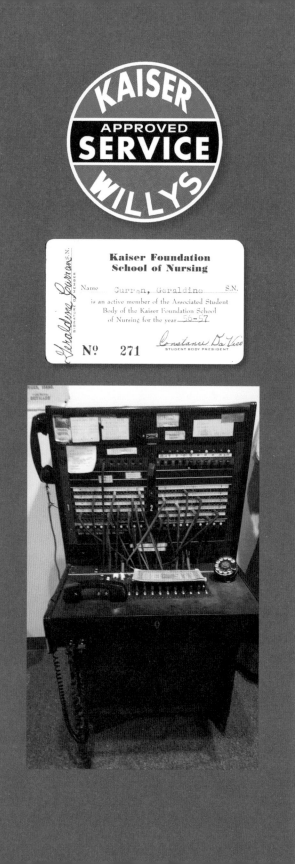

textbooks. There was even a small stipend starting with the first entering class. It started at $10 a month and increased each student year until seniors were receiving $25 — but after buying personal toiletries, white stockings and other necessities there wasn't much left for eating out, movies and discretionary spending. Some students supplemented the stipend by running the school's switchboard on the first floor (a holdover from the days when the dorm was the Piedmont Hotel). Also, during their senior year, students could choose to work in the hospital on weekends for pay and assume patient responsibilities consistent with their level of training. Faculty member Nadine Byrd also was present and served as a resource for the students working at the hospital on the weekends. The hospital work not only gave them spending money, but was an opportunity to continue learning outside of class, and it aided their transition from student to practicing RN.

In addition to the school's low tuition, scholarships were available. The experience of Janice Price

*(Top to bottom) Sign advertising a
Kaiser Willys service station c. 1954.*

Membership card.

*School telephone switchboard; managing the switchboard
was a source of extra income for students.*

Klein, class of '63, was similar to that of many entering students. "I got scholarships from three different groups: The Soroptimists, the school and from an organization of World War I veterans — 'The Forty & Eight' (40 ET 8)." These veterans were expressing their gratitude to the nursing profession for caring for them and their wounded buddies in France during The Great War. "They chose to give me money for my first year. They loved the nurses who had kept them alive. I was very blessed, really because there just was no money."[26]

The story of Helen Harrison Robinson, class of '65, was typical. She had been a member of the Future Nurses Club at Oakland High School, but she didn't think it would be financially possible for her to attend the school. The $10 application fee was a real barrier for her and her family. At a time when the purchasing power of $10 was significant, her family was able to raise it, knowing that once she was in school most of her expenses would be covered.

DIVERSITY

From the beginning, the school had a student body that was ethnically and socioeconomically diverse. While racism was far more visible and present throughout the United States, including in the Bay Area, ethnic and socioeconomic diversity already was a feature of the entire Kaiser medical care program. It was mirrored in the school faculty as well as in the makeup of the Health Plan membership which, unlike other medical institutions in the region, had been open to all races right from its inception in 1942.

Henry Kaiser and Sidney Garfield had made nondiscrimination a core value of the Kaiser continuum of medical care, and this attitude had the desired effect on the nursing school. KFSN's practice of nondiscrimination in student admissions and in consistently recruiting minority students set it apart from other nursing schools in California.

Defying the trends of discrimination and segregation endemic in the culture of the time and teaching all students equally added a layer of confidence among KFSN's African American students. This legacy of disrupting the cultural norm of discrimination had an extensive impact on nursing and patient care. Black student nurses participated in initiatives that addressed health care disparities in the black community and promoted inclusion, diversity and health equity for all patients.

This nondiscrimination approach and the school's low cost made nursing education available to many students from economically disadvantaged backgrounds who would have not been able to obtain a professional nursing education. As friendships developed, appreciating that diversity became part of the education these young women received.

The richness of diversity and the open, supportive environment encouraged the students to share with and learn from one another. One conversation that took place in the dorm one evening involved African American and Japanese American students. Juliette Whitfield Powell, class of '58, an African American student, was in her dorm room relaxing with her roommate (another black student) and with two Japanese American students. One of the Japanese Americans was Grace Oshita Miyamoto from Lahaina, Hawaii, and the other was from Penryn, a small town near Auburn in California's Sierra Mountains.

The student from California asked the Hawaiian girl where she and her family had been interned during the war. Powell and Miyamoto had no idea what the question meant. They were incredulous, asking if the California student meant she was sent to a concentration camp. The African American students had never heard of this wartime episode. The student from Penryn was equally incredulous; she had thought all Japanese Americans had been interned. Even though the Japanese attack had been in Hawaii, there had been no internment there.

Miyamoto explained to an interviewer years later that at the time she, too, had never heard about the Japanese internment that had taken place on the mainland. Now, she says, "There were so many of us that if they'd had to put us in those concentration camps, the island would sink! (laughs) That's how I handled it."[27]

As the girls from different backgrounds got to know one another in conversations like this, their horizons were widened and barriers of race and social background fell away, further unifying the student body as well as preparing them for a diverse workplace and caring for a diversity of patients.

KFSN: A RESPECTED LEADER IN NURSING EDUCATION

One goal was very clear in MacLean's mind. She wanted nothing less than for the Kaiser Foundation School of Nursing to become a respected leader in American nursing education. She recognized when she began in 1953 that she faced some unique obstacles, including the suspicion of the Health Plan held by local professionals. These professional groups ran ongoing campaigns denigrating the quality of care available through the Health Plan, and much of the general public believed their propaganda. Her approach to reaching her goal and to overcoming obstacles followed three major routes:

- Outstanding test scores
- Leadership
- Top faculty with innovative educational approaches

OUTSTANDING TEST SCORES

The first and most direct route was demonstrating the quality of the education the students received. Evidence of this showed up on the state of California's standardized tests that all nursing school graduates have to pass before they become registered nurses. During the Daniels administration, the scores certainly had been respectable, but now they began to improve class by class as new faculty members were added and the curriculum was adjusted based on the experiences of previous classes. Before long, students consistently were scoring among the top three schools in the entire state, even outperforming the more prestigious schools attached to universities.

LEADERSHIP

MacLean also had another technique for raising the school's profile in the nursing profession. Since the beginning, each class had officers. Daniels had selected Francine Weir Ammerman to be president of the first class, but each class after that elected its own president. Many early students remember how they developed leadership skills as class officers. MacLean encouraged students to reach outside of the school, to participate first in the California Nursing Students' Association (CNSA) and then to become active in the American Nursing Association. She provided funds for class and student body officers to travel to meetings of the CNSA and to the National Student Nurses' Association (NSNA).

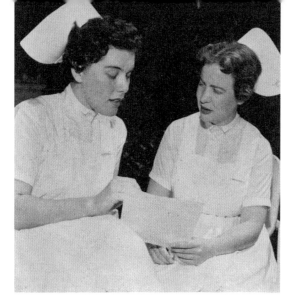

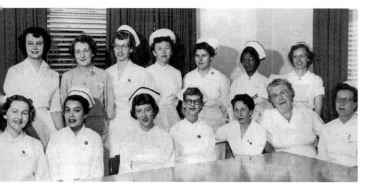

(Top to bottom) Mary Lou Steinke and classmate Phyllis Plant Moroney plan speaker bureau to reach prospective nursing students.

Faculty that developed inspiring and caring nurses through innovative teaching methods.

Many years later, Marilyn Nystrom Aiken, class of '55, president of her class, recalled it was clear to her that MacLean wanted the school to be visible and respected for the quality of nurses it produced. As president, Aiken represented KFSN at CNSA and NSNA meetings. Kaiser students Jean Berg Meddaugh, class of '57B, Carol Lyons Tribble, class of '57A, and Mary Louise Steinke Vivier, class of '57A, went to Chicago to represent the school at the annual meeting of the NSNA. Their poise and professionalism was a credit to

the school and it paid off. At that meeting, Steinke was nominated for the position of president of the national organization. The election that followed was a lively affair. Steinke supporters even had campaign buttons made up, illustrated with a cute drawing of a skunk with the catchphrase, "Don't be stinky, vote Steinke." Steinke won.

In the summer of 1957, Steinke, as the president, represented the United States' National Student Nurses' Association at the International Council of Nurses in Rome, where she was elected president of the newly organized International Student Nurses Association (today known as the International Council of Student Nursing Assembly). For the next four years, although no longer a student, Steinke held this position — the highest honor a student nurse could obtain.

Steinke's achievements and honors increased the prestige of the school. Students, faculty and people throughout the Health Plan took pride in the school's growing stature. Her election wins brought further recognition, at a national and international level, that KFSN had now taken its place as one of the most outstanding nursing schools in the country.

When Steinke returned from Chicago, she and Phyllis Plant Moroney, class of '57A, formed a speaker's bureau to reach out to students at California high schools who might be interested in a nursing education. Although their target audience was primarily sophomores who would have time to take the right courses to be eligible for admission to KFSN, they also spoke to nursing clubs at high schools to tell students already interested in a nursing career about the unique qualities of KFSN and why they should consider applying there.

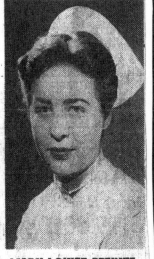

50   Oakland Tribune, Friday, June 7, 1957

Nurse at Kaiser to Head Group

Miss Mary Louise Steinke of Lafayette, a student nurse at the Kaiser Foundation School of Nursing, is the new president of the International Student Nurses Association.

She was elected at the 11th International Nursing Congress which ended Saturday in Rome, Italy. She attended the meeting as president of the American Student Nurses Association.

Miss Steinke, 22, in her new position will held a world organization of student nurses representing 71 countries.

After her graduation this month, Miss Steinke will begin her nursing career in the U.S. Navy.

She is the daughter of Navy Capt. and Mrs. Frederick Steinke of 3345 Helen Lane, Lafayette.

MARY LOUISE STEINKE
Heads World Nurse Group

Mary Steinke Named Prexy Of Nurse Unit

Miss Mary Louise Steinke, student nurse, Kaiser Foundation School of Nursing, Oakland, has been elected president of the International Student Nurses Association which convened recently in Rome, Italy.

The election was held during the final day meeting of the 11th International Nursing Congress to which Miss Steinke, who is also president of the American Student Nurses Association, was U.S. delegate.

As president of the newly-organized International Association, Miss Steinke will head a world organization of student nurses representing some 71 countries.

Miss Steinke, an attractive 22-year old blonde, will graduate this June from the Kaiser School of Nursing in Oakland, and plans to begin her nursing career in the U.S. Navy.

She is the daughter of Navy Captain and Mrs. Frederick Steinke of 3345 Helen Lane, Lafayette.

These were not to be Mary Louise Steinke Vivier's only election victories — she'd clearly learned more than nursing at KFSN. After a long nursing career that included teaching, lecturing, holding leadership positions in the medical field as well as years of civic leadership, she was elected mayor of Visalia, California. Her retirement was lauded in the U.S. Congressional Record, noting she had gone "far above the call of duty to immerse herself in the needs of others and her community."

TOP FACULTY WITH INNOVATIVE EDUCATIONAL APPROACHES

MacLean's third approach to making certain the Kaiser Foundation School of Nursing became a respected leader in American nursing education was to hire the best faculty available and give them the freedom to innovate. Marion Yeaw, a faculty member from 1953 to 1976, is one example of this approach.

Yeaw had been hired by Dorothea Daniels in 1951 to work with newborns in the hospital. As the only Permanente nurse to hold a master's degree in nursing, Yeaw became the assistant teaching supervisor in the hospital's newborn nursery. This was at the peak of the postwar baby boom. As assistant teaching supervisor, she worked with students from the nursing school, a few at a time, familiarizing them in the operation of a newborn nursery and what their responsibilities would be after graduation. She also worked one on one with new mothers, teaching them techniques for caring for their newborns. Although she experienced great satisfaction teaching, the nursery was so busy there wasn't much time for it, and after two years, she became restless. That was when she learned that the school's new director, MacLean, was hiring faculty. Yeaw applied for a teaching position. Although she had little experience teaching, her educational background and obvious enthusiasm for teaching were enough to convince MacLean to hire her as an instructor in pediatrics.

Yeaw was grateful for the opportunity but slightly intimidated with her new role because she had never taught students in a classroom. MacLean quickly reassured her she was always available if she needed advice or help.[28]

Yeaw was in the right place. Twenty years before organizational consultants were recommending it, Marguerite MacLean was encouraging the school's faculty to experiment with their educational approach, in what decades later would be called "thinking outside the box." MacLean even went one step further. She understood that if you have a truly innovative organization, failures are inevitable. Yeaw described how it had worked in her case:

"I would get an idea and I would call her up. She'd say, 'C'mon over.' I'd go over it with her. Maybe she'd make a couple of suggestions, then [say] 'OK, Go ahead.' Sometimes it worked and I reported back that it had worked, and sometimes it didn't work. ..."[29]

If the idea did not work out, MacLean did not react by reprimanding, but emphasized what had been learned in the attempt.

"She listened to me," Yeaw said. "I told her what I had tried. I'd had objectives worked out. She said, 'I wanted to tell you, when you were telling me, that it wouldn't work, but I knew you would be so disappointed if you didn't get a chance to try. It wouldn't be right. ... Besides ... it might have.'"

Yeaw had been particularly struck by that last sentence, "It might have." MacLean was encouraging experimentation. By not insisting on 100 percent success, she opened the door for the faculty to innovate.

During the early 1950s, the California State Board of Nurse Examiners, today's California Board of Registered Nursing, began encouraging nursing schools to incorporate psycho-social factors into their curricula. This was during the time when Arnold Gesell at Yale and pediatrician/author Benjamin Spock were transforming the ideas of child growth and development. Yeaw found the developing field fascinating, and MacLean gave her the freedom to do something about it. Yeaw designed an innovative 18-hour course for the nursing students. "I set up a program where each student spent a week playing with the patients, the babies, and with whoever was there," Yeaw recalled.[30]

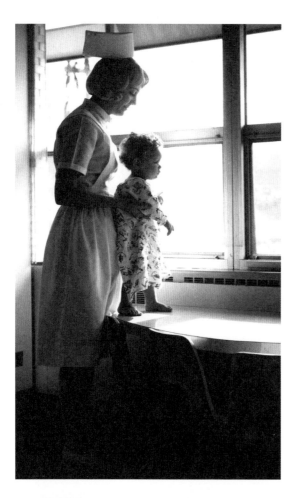

Yeaw wanted the students to compare their observations of their pediatric patients' developmental milestones, such as sitting up and crawling, with what they saw in textbooks. She knew her students wouldn't have time to go through all the textbooks themselves, so she did it for them.

"I went through all the reference books of the research that had been done of growth and development," she said. "No two agreed on any one particular age. One book would say that babies sit up at six months; another would say four and a half months. I kind of averaged them out and put the average down in what I called 'The Manual.' It was about 4–5 pages long. Each student got one that she could keep. She could fill in places here and there for the ages. It gave them something solid. If they read different books, they'd get confused. I thought that when they hit the state boards, it would give them a number so that if they'd see a number that was slightly different, they could still answer the question correctly. And it worked."[31]

(Top to bottom) Student shows pediatric patient the view outside the window.

Student describing her patient assessment to the instructor.

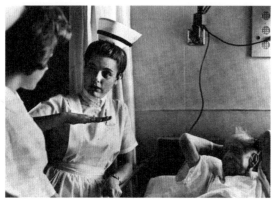

Soon after this, Yeaw took a course in growth and development at San Francisco State University. She brought to class a copy of the manual she had prepared. "One of the fellows sitting next to me said, 'Where did you get that?' I told him I wrote it. He looked at me as though I was crazy. Imagine a woman accomplishing anything like that. I said, 'I'll give you a copy of it.' It said Kaiser Foundation School of Nursing across the top!"[32]

THE ROLE OF ACADEMICS

The relationship between classroom teaching and experiences on the hospital ward was carefully designed to give students the opportunity to utilize what they had learned in the classroom and apply it to patients. It was a hallmark of the school's educational approach, details of which were evaluated continually by the faculty. Improvements were made and then re-evaluated again and again in a continuing effort to improve teaching methods. However, the nursing school was not equipped to provide the academic courses needed to fully round out students' education. For courses in such disciplines as anatomy, microbiology and physiology, the students were enrolled in and commuted to local colleges, including College of the Holy Names and Contra Costa Community College. In addition to lessons learned in these college classrooms, there were some unplanned benefits.

Many students remember the commuting camaraderie when they would joke, commiserate about academic challenges, share life experiences and sing. These trips became one more way for students to bond and form enduring friendships.

In their college classes they met students from the nursing schools at Highland and Samuel Merritt hospitals who were taking the same junior college courses. While they often made friends, the Kaiser students were pleased to point out their accommodations in the converted hotel provided them with the privacy and convenience of double rooms, each with its own bathroom, rather than dormitory-style living with communal bathrooms. More importantly, as Kaiser graduate Phyllis Plant Moroney, class of '57A, recalls:

"Everybody looked down on us as though we were some sort of guttersnipes because it (Kaiser) was 'socialized medicine' and other 'bad' things. We really had to battle out in the public about this. However, we knew from going out to the junior colleges for our academic studies that we knew far more than the other nursing students because we'd been trained differently."[33]

Originally, when the students took community college courses, they, along with students from the Highland, Providence and Samuel Merritt nursing schools, were enrolled in classes designed especially for nursing students. Courses required for a nursing diploma such as biology, chemistry, physiology and anatomy actually were watered-down versions of the academic courses also offered by the schools to their academic students. For completing each of these special nursing courses, a student received two credits toward her RN diploma — but there was a catch. Those credits were not transferable toward an associate of arts (AA) degree.

However, those college students who completed the academic version of these courses received three credits toward an AA degree. MacLean realized this put KFSN graduates who wanted to continue their education at a major disadvantage.

They would have to take these same courses over, this time in their full academic version. MacLean insisted the Kaiser students, unlike students from the other area hospital-based nursing schools, take the more rigorous courses that offered full academic credit.

This change had dual implications: Firstly, the students were better prepared to understand the "why," not just the "how" or "what" of their training. This enhanced their capacity for critical thinking, which was a key aspect of how the students were taught. Clair O'Sullivan Lisker, class of '51, who later joined the faculty, remembers how she would "drill" students on the floor of the wards with questions such as, "Why are you doing what you are doing; what is the reason behind it? Why are you weighing the patient every morning? Why are you measuring the patient's urine? Have you checked the results of the tests the patient had yesterday?" She wanted them to understand the meaning behind the care they were giving the patient. "I would ask them questions," she said. "'Give me the reasons you are doing what you are doing. You need to know that.'"[34]

Secondly, KFSN students could see in their faculty women who demonstrated the opportunities

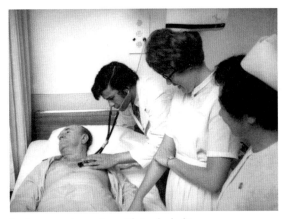
Students assessing patient with faculty looking on.

and advantages available to nurses with advanced educations. Having those academic credits that counted toward a college degree was another encouragement for students to continue their education after graduating from Kaiser.

In 1967, the school became the first diploma nursing program in California to offer a junior college associate of arts in nursing degree. In so doing, KFSN also was responding to a movement within the nursing profession toward college-based classroom work and supervised clinical internships. This later would have important implications for the school's future.

MacLean's own relationship with the students was a complex one. To many students, she was a towering authoritarian figure. Lynn DeForest Robie,

class of '57B, who was there when MacLean took over from Daniels, said of the two: "They both were tough, you really had to behave. But Miss MacLean was of another school. She really, really cared about us and you were going to learn — or else."[35]

Other students remembered MacLean's classes covering her very definite ideas about how the students should act and dress when not in uniform, and what makeup was appropriate. She was determined that students and graduates would well represent the school and the Kaiser name. Jean Berg Meddaugh, class of '57B, remembered, "She was very stern about the way you acted, how you addressed people, your appearance, all those values." Other faculty members reinforced MacLean's "social" lessons, but the real impetus came from the top, from MacLean herself.[36]

On the other hand, Meddaugh also recalled another side of MacLean. When Meddaugh had been elected president of the student body, "One of the things I had to do was to give a speech in a ceremony for the younger students who were receiving their caps. I wrote the speech and I was ill one day. Miss MacLean came in person to check on me and asked me to share my speech with her. I remember how nice she was, how encouraging she was."[37]

TEAM LEADERSHIP

Another way students developed the leadership ability that would distinguish KFSN graduates was to work as team leaders. Aiken, who several years after graduating from KFSN joined the faculty, described how it worked from her perspective as a supervising instructor: "A senior would be a team leader. She would have maybe three people working under her taking care of a group of patients. When I was on the floor supervising, I would work with the senior team leader, tell her what I was interested in and get her feedback on the younger students that she was responsible for."[38]

Later in her career, Marilyn Nystrom Aiken, class of '55, became a hospital administrator grateful for the leadership skills she developed as a student. "I needed to be good at organizing, to be a good speaker. I gave a lot of speeches. ... It all started with that student responsibility."[39]

As team leader, the senior student was developing her leadership skills by overseeing the work of younger students who were caring for a total of perhaps 30 patients. Sylvia Barnes Bertram, class of '64, described her experience of leading a care team while a student, and what it meant to her:

"You averaged 28 to 30 patients. There were no coronary care units, no intensive care units. You had a mix of patients and you were responsible for all the IVs and all the medications and coordinating with the people who took their vital signs, bathed them. We had RNs and LVNs and maybe five aides. I remember that I was overwhelmed by the number of patients. That seemed like a lot because when you go on clinical as a student, you have two patients. Later that seemed to be a piece of cake."

She went on to reflect how that realization shaped her career. "Wasn't long after I graduated from school that I became aware that nursing was the profession for me, not a job. Those are two very different things. ... I believe that the words were used at the nursing school but the words never sunk in the way they did when I was surrounded by people who treated it as a job. They had gone to other schools. I think the foundation of my feelings came out of the nursing program. It isn't just a job. It deals with real people and you influence them."[40]

During MacLean's administration, students' grades had improved until they rivaled and then began to exceed the performance of more established schools. It was becoming increasingly clear that the KFSN approach to nursing education, where students' clinical exposure was built around their educational needs rather than hospital staffing needs, was bringing excellent results.

During this period, the school's overall dropout rate remained at about 50 percent between freshman enrollment and graduation. Most students left during the first months. However, once a student was accepted into the school, faculty members continued to do whatever they could, without lowering standards, to help her, (and later him), complete the course. They often gave generously of their own time to do it. Aiken recalled, with justifiable pride, the experience of one of her students. The year before, this student had failed the six-month probation period but had been allowed to return to the school for a second chance. Her instructors had passed her in her other courses. Aiken would be the last to weigh in on whether this student should be allowed to continue at KFSN, and she had her doubts. This student's future in nursing was looking bleak. "I ended up as her last chance," Aiken recalled. "I could see that she was terrified of authority, so I worked with her through my senior team leader. I had her assign the student to patients in the beds furthest from the door. ... and I could sneak into the room and listen to what she was doing with the patient. I did that all the time that she was on my floor."

Then it was time for Aiken to make a decision about this student's future.

"I scheduled a conference with her and we went to the empty dining room. I remember I was sitting across the table from her. I reviewed her experience and at the end I told her that I was approving her to go on. I'll never forget this, she looked at me, dumbfounded, and she said, 'You are the only person who has ever believed in me.'"[41]

That student went on to graduate. A few years later, Aiken was approached by one of the nurses who'd been a classmate of the student at the nursing school. "She asked me, 'Do you know who the evening supervisor at the hospital is?' It was that same student, who came so close to being dropped from the school but who, with Aiken's encouragement, had finished and was now a nursing supervisor. Aiken finished the anecdote on a note of pride. "That's a story I have never forgotten."[42]

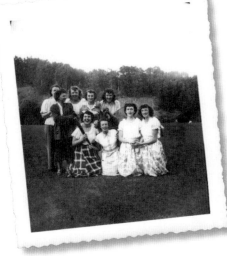

KFSN NURSES' REPUTATION WITH PHYSICIANS

KFSN graduates soon earned the respect of the physicians they worked with. Ron Bachman, MD, a leading Permanente physician, recalled, "All I know is that it was common among the Permanente physicians that if the nurse had gone to our nursing school, we could trust her more, we could know that she knew her way around, and we were just more comfortable with them and felt they worked out better."[43]

When asked what made KFSN nurses better than graduates from other programs, he referred to the kind of training they had received. "As a group, they were smart, they were practical and they trained with us," he said. The doctors understood that it made a difference in their practice that these nurses had been trained in a prepaid group practice where there was an emphasis on teamwork, patient education and prevention.[44]

Students, too, recognized the unique value of their KFSN education. Naomi Eiko Tanikawa, class of '54A, wrote a remarkably prescient prediction in the student publication, "The Drawsheet," in 1953: "We believe the day will come when KFSN will be recognized as one of the leaders in progressive nursing education."[45]

Marguerite MacLean had come to Kaiser to lead what was already a top-quality nursing school, graduating nurses who already were prepared to step into their new profession. She had led the school into a period of growth and innovation. With KFSN students' consistently high test scores on the nursing boards as well as word-of-mouth evaluations from physicians and co-workers, the school's reputation for excellence spread throughout the nursing profession. According to TPMG physician and historian John Smillie, "The school was now enriching the Permanente organization with an appreciation and respect for the profession of nursing as an essential component of group practice."[46]

(Above) Students outdoor trip.

(Opposite) Drawsheet, by and for the students of Kaiser Foundation School of Nursing.

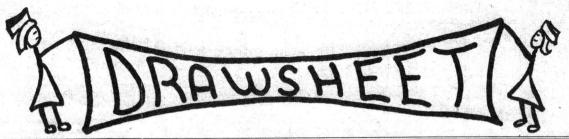

DRAWSHEET

Volume II, No. 1   OCTOBER, 1953   Oakland, California

The East Bay Student Nurses Association

For the benefit of the girls who are uninformed on the functions of the East Bay Student Nurse Association: It is an organization of the four East Bay nursing schools formed to promote better inter-school relationships by group discussions and social functions such as the annual spring formal, which was held at the Mira Vista Country club last year.

Each school has an official representative who is requested to be present at all the meetings, and present a summary to the student body.

A meeting was held at Providence Hospital October 15, 1953, and the California State Student Nurse Convention was discussed. The convention this year will be held in San Francisco on November 19 and 20. All students are cordially invited to attend. There is a registration fee of $1.50. Transportation will be furnished to and from the meetings. There will be a dinner held November 19, also open to all students, with a charge of $4.75 a plate.

Kaiser Foundation student body will be represented at the convention by Misses Jessie Head, Student body president; Emily Mitchell, E.B.S.N.A. representative, and Ellie White, State representative. Jan Bartels, president of E.B.S.N.A. will be jointly sponsored by the four schools.

A poster contest on the subject of recruitment of student nurses is being sponsored at present with the winning poster to be on display at the convention. Details may be obtained from Ellie White, room 314.

An anniversary paper will be published for the convention if all the schools approve a five dollar pledge for 50 copies. The issue will contain pictures and articles on the speakers and the other highlights of the convention.

At the last student body meeting a motion was passed to donate five dollars to the newly organized National Student Nurses Association.

The next meeting of the E.B.S. N.A. will be held at Highland on the second Tuesday of November. Kaiser should have a larger representation in the future than we have in the past so let's all plan to attend.

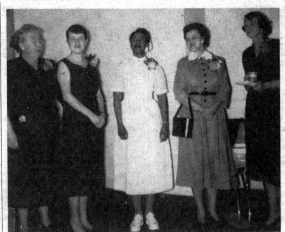

From left to right, Miss MacLean, L. Oyarzo, J. Head, Miss Convelski, Miss McFarland.

Last Friday, October 16, an informal tea was given honoring the presence of our new Assistant Director of Nursing Education, Miss Stephanie Convelski, and Miss McFarland, our new Medical Social Worker. The tea was held in the dining room from 3:00 until 4:30. A large number of the staff and many students attended.

In the receiving line were the guests of honor: Miss Jessie Head, president of the student body; Miss LaVerne Oyarzo, president of the senior class, and Miss Marguerite MacLean, Director of the School of Nursing. We were also honored by the presence of Miss M. Cam-

eron and Mrs. J. Boernge, members of the State Board of Nurse Examiners.

Tea was poured by Mrs. Wilson, social worker, and coffee was served by our house mother, Mrs. Reese. The tables were elaborately decorated with chrysanthemums of brilliant fall colors.

A note of recognition for those wonderful hors d'oeuvres made by the pre-clinical class. Many compliments were heard about them, floating around the room between gulps and smiles.

It has been heard that many more teas are to be held in the future for our experience. Hope everyone takes full advantage of it.

Plans for Christmas Formal Commence Date Set Dec. 19

Plans are being made for the annual Christmas formal. This year's dance promises to be better than ever. Reservations have been made at the Sequoia Country Club for Saturday, December 19, 1953, from 9 p.m. to 1 a.m. Most of you will remember this is where we had our Christmas Dance last year. Tentative committees have been appointed. They are: Miss Paddock in charge of obtaining an orchestra; N. Tanikawa, bids; H. Scheuermann, decorations; P. Simmons, advertisement. Bids will go on sale December 2.

Card Party Sponsored By Drawsheet Staff

The Drawsheet Staff is sponsoring a card party Wednesday, November 4, 1953, to be held in the penthouse of the nurses' residence from 6:30 p.m. until 10 o'clock p.m. A charge of 25c shall be made to each contestant. The following games will be offered: chess, checkers, four handed canasta, pinochle, and bridge. Prizes will be given to the winners and a booby prize to those of us who have lost our beginners' luck. Refreshments consisting of coffee and cookies will be served. Choose a pardner, challenge your best friends, and get out the cards to practice. We'll see all of you in the penthouse.

Mrs. E. Henshaw Executive Sect. School of Nursing

Among the many new personalities seen around Kaiser School of Nursing is the very pleasant Mrs. Henshaw.

She may be found in her office on the third floor where she carries out her duties as Executive Secretary to the School of Nursing and Social Advisor to the students.

Previously, Mrs. Henshaw was associated with Miss Daniels and in September of this year, assumed her present position.

A native of Oakland, Mrs. Henshaw graduated from the U.C. with a B.A. degree. She is the mother of two children, a boy age 9 and a girl age 11. Her favorite sport is swimming, and gardening is listed as her favorite hobby.

As our social advisor Mrs. Henshaw states she will be glad to give advice and help students with their problems.

We are proud and happy to have Mrs. Henshaw with us and extend her a very hearty welcome.

The Seniors Speak

A recent cause for loud protest on the part of the seniors was the suggestion that students who reached the 18 month mark in their nursing course be allowed to wear their black bands on their caps. It is generally felt among both seniors and lower classmen, that wearing the black bands marks the "beginning of the end." Like capping, it is a goal to which we work and a cause for rejoicing when the last six months is reached. So, unless something unforeseen occurs, black bands will remain the strict property of the high seniors.

As soon as the class pins arrive, they will appear on the caps of the seniors. The pin is diamond-shaped with a Caduceus as the motif, and connected by a chain to a lamp. It is gold with black etching and has the year "1954" engraved on the lamp.

Greetings to the Probies

We, of the outgoing senior class, wish to extend a welcome to the incoming class of 1956-B. We know 1956 sounds an eternity away, but the years slip by all too soon and soon 1956 will be upon you.

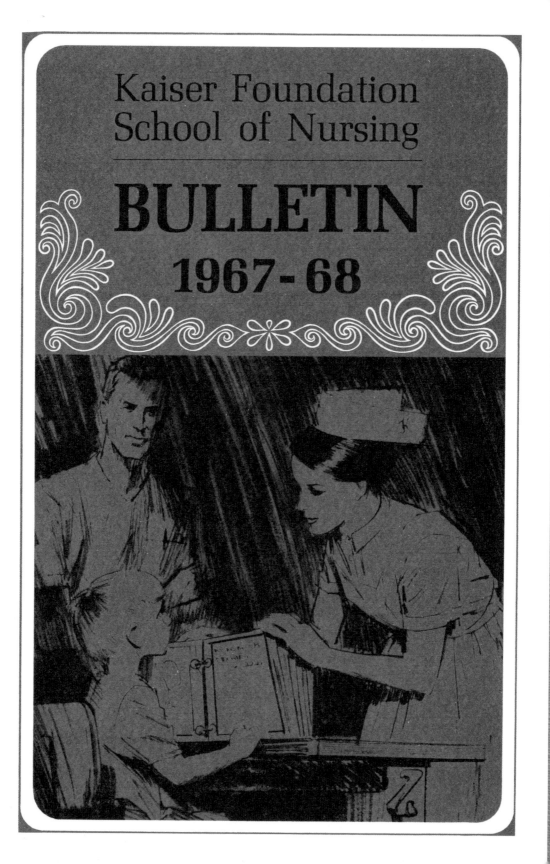

Kaiser Foundation
School of Nursing

BULLETIN
1967- 68

the COPPEDGE ERA

SELF-CARE. NURSING LEADERSHIP. PUBLIC POLICY **4** DIVERSITY. MALE NURSES. PATIENT-CENTERED CARE

The 1960s and 1970s

BY 1957 MARGUERITE MACLEAN HAD MANY REASONS TO FEEL SATISFIED. After taking over from Dorothea Daniels, she'd broken away from traditional norms and successfully transformed the school into a model of innovative nursing education never seen or imagined before. She guided its transition from a hospital-based nursing school organized along the standard nursing educational lines of the time to a school that no longer was a subsidiary of a hospital. While so doing, she also redirected its primary purpose away from patient care and toward the education of its students.

The Kaiser Foundation School of Nursing was now a freestanding, high-caliber educational institution ranked among the best in California. She decided it was time for her to think about retirement.

Aware of MacLean's decision, the Kaiser Foundation Board of Trustees selected a new director, Josephine Coppedge. She was well prepared for the responsibility of directing the school. She had received a bachelor's degree in nursing education from San Jose State College and a master's degree in nursing service administration from the University of Colorado. MacLean agreed to stay on for several months to smooth the transition, allowing Josephine Coppedge to begin to put her own mark on the school.

THE JOSEPHINE COPPEDGE ERA BEGINS

Decades later, student memories of Josephine Coppedge are remarkably vivid. Despite being short in stature, Coppedge was an imposing figure who carried herself with a military bearing, no doubt a result of the years she had spent in the U.S. Army Nurse Corps.

It immediately became clear to the students that the new director saw herself as their role model. Bea Rudney, who had joined the faculty as health director for the students in the late 1960s, recalled, "She had tight reins on how they looked and how they behaved. She put a lot of emphasis on appearance, on posture. She even had classes with them on posture. That was important to her."[1]

Lesley Meriwether, class of '63, described the director's attitude from a student perspective: "Mrs. Coppedge was very direct about what she expected from us. She asked direct questions. She was not a chummy person; [she was] much more formal. She told you what she expected of you. If she had an interview with you, she was very much to the point."[2]

Meriwether compared the role of the school director in students' lives with that of the school's 24 faculty members, which now included a librarian, counselor and health nurse: "She was not a professor. Our nursing professors were very friendly with us and were very supportive directly," Meriwether noted. "They would hug us if we needed it. That was not [Coppedge's] kind of thing. She was a formal person. She did the business part of things. She was the front. What things looked like was very important to her."[3]

While the director did not teach nursing classes, the students saw her in a classroom, where she taught them the specifics of how to create and maintain the image she believed was essential to being a truly professional nurse. This included how a student should arrange her hair, do her makeup, walk and dress. Coppedge was "always dressed very beautifully, very thoughtfully," Meriwether recalled. She said Coppedge's hair was done, her nails were done, and that she always looked very nice. She set "very high standards for how you handled yourself, how you were to wear makeup (if you wore any)."[4]

To Gretchen Mueller Seifert, class of '59, "Mrs. Coppedge was a lovely person, although a bit formidable. I always liked her. I thought she had a really tough job, and I don't think she was given her due by many students. I don't think she was cherished by all students, but I liked her a lot. I think she was a wise woman."[5]

Elizabeth Ann Miller Moore, class of '60, who years later became an instructor of medicine/ surgery at KFSN, recalled a class taught by Coppedge: "It was called Professional Adjustment. It was about how to sit, stand, walk; how to do your nails. Whenever we went out, we had to wear hats and gloves, because that was what you did in the Bay Area in those days. You did not go into the city, San Francisco, without wearing a hat and gloves."[6] There even was a reference book titled "The Nurse's Guide to Beauty, Charm, Poise" that acknowledged KFSN on the title page. This book went as far as giving instructions on how to smoke like a lady.[7]

Moore went on to say, "The only thing Mrs. Coppedge ever yelled at me for was because I'd run up and down the hall and into the office and, this is a quote, 'Elizabeth Ann, put on your shoes. You are liable to step on a thumbtack.' My

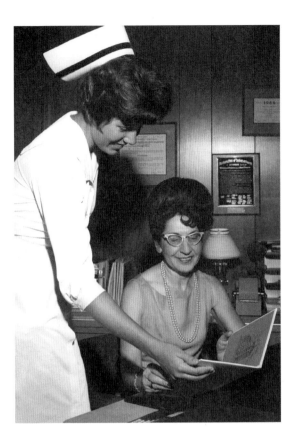

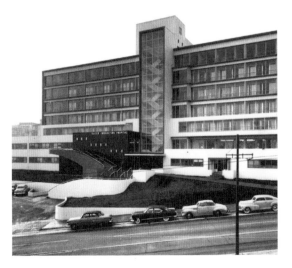

(Top to bottom) Mrs. Coppedge and graduating student.

San Francisco Kaiser Hospital c. 1954.

parents happened to be there at that time. After that, my father would continually remind me, 'Elizabeth Ann, put on your shoes!'"[8]

Rebecca Schoenthal Calloway, class of '61, said it seemed that sometimes Coppedge went to extremes: "At our little meetings, she would tell us how to iron our shoelaces so we would look good, and tell us that Kaiser girls [should] never take off their shoes at dances we had with fraternities at Stanford and UC Berkeley, or at the Merchant Marine Academy."[9]

Another student told of Coppedge checking the lengths of their skirts before she would let them go to work in the hospital. She would direct them to kneel, and if the hem of a uniform did not reach the floor, the student would be sent back to her room to dress properly.

According to Kristin Weaver, class of '73, there was also a bit of "do as I say, not as I do" to Coppedge. She remembers looking out of a residence window overlooking the parking lot and seeing the school's director get into her pink Cadillac. Then, the woman who told her students never to smoke in public lit a cigarette and drove away with it dangling from her mouth.[10]

For Coppedge, "teaching moments" could come at any time. One evening, at a dinner celebrating a class reaching an important milestone, she was seated next to Deloras Plake Jones, class of '63. Coppedge took this as an opportunity to teach the young student how to eat chicken properly.[11]

Coppedge shared her predecessor's belief in the importance of KFSN graduates being not only well trained in their profession, but also expanding their interests to help them enjoy a well-rounded life.

Despite finding requirements such as ironed shoelaces silly and a bit annoying, Rebecca Schoenthal Calloway was quick to credit Coppedge with sparking her lifelong interest in theater and music by arranging for students to travel to San Francisco for concerts, plays and musicals. KFSN's previous director, Dorothea Daniels, believed in cultivating interests outside of nursing as a form of self-care. Underscoring and presciently forecasting self-care as an essential antidote to burnout, Daniels wrote an American Journal of Nursing article in 1940 describing the importance of self-care for nursing students, which resulted in her making it a part of the students' education.[12]

MacLean had agreed with Daniels and provided continued enrichment and growth opportunities for students outside the school. This promotion of the value of self-care through developing outside recreational activities had continued into the current environment; Coppedge was carrying on what had become a tradition going back to the earliest days of the school. Calloway is just one of the many KFSN graduates who think this exposure to the arts, which led to new lifelong interests, helped her and other graduates avoid burnout later in their careers. Coppedge also reminded students that they were at all times representing the school of nursing.

Once a month, the student body met with the director. Topics ranged from updates about what was going on in the hospital, such as personnel changes and staff reassignments that might affect the students' clinical experience, to items directly related to the students. For example, an incident was raised of a student who had been seen speeding across the Bay Bridge to San Francisco driving the school's station wagon to the Kaiser Hospital. Students were reminded that when driving, as everywhere else, they were representing the school.

In an article that appeared in the KP Reporter, an in-house publication for Kaiser Permanente employees, Judy Wilson Fiebelkorn, class of '63, described the activities Coppedge encouraged students to engage in to fill their "free" time. These activities offered many opportunities for developing leadership skills and habits. One example was the Big and Little Sister Program, in which the older students took responsibility for helping the incoming freshmen to adjust to school life in the dormitory and in the classroom. This, too, often was the beginning of an enduring friendship.

Students who lived near the school often would invite a classmate or friend home for the weekend. They would bring back food their mothers had prepared. One of these students was Helen Harrison Robinson, class of '65, an African American student from Oakland. Her mother would send them back to school with a traditional family Sunday supper, while other parents sent students back with such ethnic treats as Japanese sushi and Filipino lumpia. These foods from home led to sharing family stories and traditions, encouraged understanding of diversity and became an enriching experience further preparing the students for practice in multiethnic institutions.

LEARNING TO BECOME NURSE LEADERS

The students were encouraged to participate in an active student council with elected officers. The student body president, and often the class president, continued the practice begun by MacLean to attend the National Student Nurses' Association convention, providing an excellent opportunity for leadership growth.

There were monthly formal and informal social affairs, where students learned to plan social events and develop skills on how to be gracious hostesses. Additionally, other student activities such as church clubs, a school paper, a choir, a yearbook, a library committee and a symphony committee offered opportunities for the young women to develop leadership skills along with their nursing studies while promoting self-care through diversion.

One of the school's signature legacies in nursing education — and a major goal of the three-year KFSN curriculum — was preparing students to be leaders in their nursing practices. In their senior year, each student experienced being a team leader in the patient care units of the hospital by leading a team of juniors on the nursing floor. As team leader, she would have two to four students working under her taking care of a small group of patients. Although there was an RN supervising the team leader, the team leader's responsibility was real, and an important step in her preparation for the responsibilities she soon would be given in what they called "the real world."

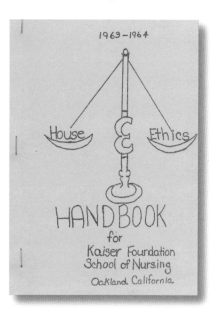

Lynn DeForest Robie, class of '57B, always appreciated the responsibility students were given as undergraduates and how well that prepared her and her classmates to begin work efficiently and effectively as registered nurses: "Before we finished school, we became the head nurse and had other nurses under us. We worked on PMs (evening shift), we worked on nights. We knew all the shifts. You don't see that in the schools today. It doesn't exist."[13]

In an interview that appeared in the August 1959 KP Reporter, Coppedge explained that the school's goal was "to train students for bedside nursing of a high caliber, caring for the total needs of a patient." In that article, Coppedge explained that she thought a nurse functioned better with the patient if she, the nurse, had a broad knowledge of human relations. She went on to say that she endeavored to enable her students, through a varied program of study and activities, to acquire such knowledge.

Eight years later, in a 1967 issue of the KP Reporter, Coppedge described how she and the faculty had further refined the direction of the school: "Our philosophy is to direct all of our efforts toward the welfare of the patient. Caring for people is what motivates most women who choose a nursing career. Others with a greater interest in teaching or administration are suited for supervisory positions. We educate both kinds of nurses at our school, because both are needed in the profession."

COMMITTEES AND COPPEDGE'S COMMITMENT TO RESOURCES AND THE FACULTY

The faculty created a variety of different student committees to deal with specific issues related to academics, lifestyle choices and ethics. One was the House and Ethics Committee. Ann Moore, class of '60, recalled: "I was on that committee, which meant focusing on discipline and health issues in the

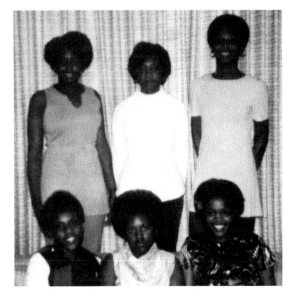

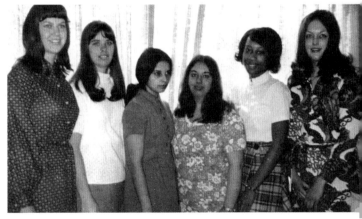

(Left to right) Kaiser students establishing a chapter of the Black Nurses Association in 1972.

Presidents/chairs of student organizations... learning to be leaders.

dorm, arrangements for graduations and so forth. We also made sure that the girls were not disobeying the rules about drinking, smoking [and] getting pregnant."[14]

Mary Louise Mott, a longtime faculty member who taught med/surg nursing and anatomy classes, explained that at faculty meetings they could make requests for whatever books, journal subscriptions, supplies and the like they thought they needed for their classes. She remembered one of her requests and how it was handled.

"We could request anything. I was doing classes on the kidney and I wanted a model kidney to show and I got one, immediately," she said. The faculty appreciated Coppedge's close relationship with the Kaiser Foundation Board, which continued to be very supportive of the nursing school. "Any time Mrs. Coppedge requested something, she got it!," Mott pointed out with appreciation, because Coppedge not only obtained all the books, equipment and facilities requested, "she even got raises for the faculty."[15]

JOSEPHINE COPPEDGE'S NATIONAL LEADERSHIP ROLES

Recognition of KFSN's continuing educational success earned Coppedge the opportunity to take on leadership roles in national professional organizations, further spreading the influence of the school in shaping public policy across the nation. She modeled the aspiration and expectation that KFSN had for its students to excel, and be visionaries and leaders in their profession. In 1967, Coppedge was appointed by U.S. Secretary of Health, Education and Welfare John Gardner to the Program Review Committee for the Nurse Training Act of 1964. This act was the most comprehensive and important nursing legislation in American history to date, and was designed to increase the nation's supply of qualified nurses by providing financial assistance to schools and students of professional nursing. The purpose of the committee was to review and study the accomplishments and frame recommendations related to the future role of government in nursing education.[16]

As appreciation of KFSN's achievements continued to spread through the profession, in 1968 Coppedge was elected to the Governing Council of the American Hospital Association's Assembly of Hospital

Schools of Nursing. The assembly represented 360 hospital schools of nursing across America and was organized to promote and improve nursing education within hospitals.[17]

She also was appointed by the National League for Nursing to the National Steering Committee for Diploma Schools of Nursing, one of the most influential groups for setting trends and policies in nursing education in the United States. KFSN increasingly was becoming recognized nationally and internationally as a leader in nursing education; Coppedge was named one of Two Thousand Women of Achievement for 1970.[18]

FACULTY ACHIEVEMENTS

Although the director headed the school, the faculty took on an increasingly important role in creating the curriculum. At weekly meetings faculty members continually were evaluating the curriculum, looking for innovations that might lead to additional improvements in educational outcomes. Clair Lisker, a graduate and then faculty member, said they had independence to choose what to teach to students and how to teach the selected information, with lively discussion among the faculty over the ideas to be taught.

Ann Moore was an instructor in medicine/surgery and a participant in those meetings. "We discussed the progress of students, of the problem students, and curriculum changes," she said. "We did a lot of talking about what we needed to do to upgrade to keep accreditation, business things."[19]

Gail Sinquefeld, who also taught medicine/surgery, described the democratic decision-making process that went on at their meetings: "We were a hardworking faculty. Sometimes people would not agree on something, but what I have to say is ... ultimately, whatever the problems, we were there trying to benefit the school and the students. Eventually, we would all be able to either agree or compromise."[20]

Asked for an example, Cynthia Reed, a faculty member who taught obstetrics, described what this freedom in curriculum development could mean to an instructor: "We worked very closely with the administration, [which] gave us the flexibility to try new innovative things. We had a teaching team

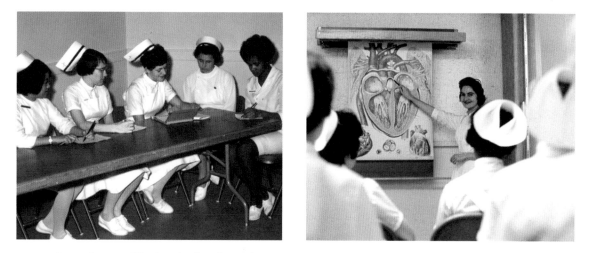

set up for each year. The head of each teaching team would report to the administration. Helen Ross was the dean of instruction, so she was the one who was most familiar with what was going on with teaching. We had more flexibility (than other schools), so I was able to do some innovative things there that weren't usually done when students spent time on the floor (clinicals). Faculty members in other specialties were doing kind of the same thing."[21]

"An example of this is in obstetrics, [where] we had a set number of weeks, eight. The students would have theory classes two days a week and clinical three days a week," she said. "I turned it around so we had four weeks of theory so that they would know a little bit of what they were doing before they even got on the floor, and then four straight weeks of clinical. It was a more concentrated kind of experience."

Another change initiated by the faculty's Curriculum Committee involved using the Kaiser San Francisco Hospital for clinicals. The faculty agreed the hospital, with its baby-in-the-drawer and other innovations, offered an opportunity to improve OB/GYN and neonatal training, so students began commuting from Oakland to San Francisco for their obstetrics rotation.

Grace Oshita Miyamoto, a member of one of the first groups of Kaiser students to be assigned to the hospital, remembered not only the hospital but also the commute: "They had the latest thing, babies in

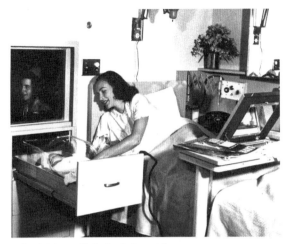

(Above) Mom calls for her baby-in-a-drawer.

(Opposite left to right) Students meeting
with instructor Clair Lisker.

Instructor Margaret Emery lecturing
on cardiac conditions.

that little drawer, rooming in. The school had a station wagon. We all got into it with Mrs. Eleanor Smith, our instructor. She was great fun. I think there were five or six of us who commuted in that station wagon every morning."[22]

Preparing the students to be teachers themselves continued as a top priority. Reed already had worked for several years at the Kaiser Oakland Hospital before deciding she really wanted to teach at the nursing school. There, she focused not only on teaching the students, but on helping those students learn to teach their patients. "Patient teaching was an important part of our curriculum,"

she said. "Along with the physical care, patient education was a big part of care given to patients."[23]

Miyamoto described it: "They wanted us to have the experience of teaching the mothers how to bathe the baby. It was interesting having us 18- and 19-year-old women teaching these mothers, but nobody thought anything strange about it. I really think the patients enjoyed having young nurses there."[24]

VALUING DIVERSITY

Over the next years, the faculty noticed that fewer ethnic minorities were applying to the school. The student body was becoming less diverse and the faculty was determined to do something about this. Faculty members traveled to high schools in northern California to speak with any young women interested in a nursing career. Marian Treter Feinstein, class of '63, remembers her experiences as a student accompanying faculty on these recruitment meetings. Because it was important that the young women who might be interested in nursing take appropriate courses early enough so they would be eligible to apply to KFSN, the faculty-student recruiters spoke to high school sophomores and juniors. Many of the students were attending schools with Future

Nurses Clubs run by the school nurse. There, students might learn some basic nursing skills, such as how to take a temperature and how to make up a hospital bed. It wasn't serious training, but it gave them a taste of what nursing might be like for them.

Clair Lisker was one of the active recruiters of minority students. "We went to the black organizations to see if we could recruit black students," Lisker recalled. "Later, we wanted to admit more students with a Mexican background – Chicanos was the term we were using. We went to Mexican organizations to see if we could interview some potential students."[25]

Their efforts soon began to pay off with a more diverse student body. In 1970, the school also began a minority scholarship program. Four Oakland high school seniors, chosen by Oakland school counselors, were awarded the scholarships. They covered 80 percent of the direct costs of the three-year program.

Around this same time, the idea of broadening diversity by enrolling men in the nursing program was coming up more frequently in faculty meetings. Although the idea of male nurses was an unusual concept for most Americans, it was not for Lisker, who had begun her nursing education in England. "We [the faculty] wanted to recruit men," Lisker said. "I was very used to having men as nurses in England. We would talk about it and thought we really needed it."[26]

Jeff Purtle, class of '74, didn't know any of this. He had been an Army medical corpsman in combat in Vietnam and also had worked with a number of nurse anesthetists in the Army's hospitals. He thought their work interesting as well as valuable, and since the Army nurse anesthetists where he was working were all male, nursing did not seem like a strange ambition, especially to be a nurse anesthetist. When his Army hitch was up, Purtle came to San Francisco. Because of his experience as an Army medic, he soon was hired as an operating room technician at Oakland's Peralta Hospital.

Oakland Tribune   Sat., May 2, 1970

Four Oakland high school girls are recipients of new minority scholarships initiated by Kaiser Foundation School of Nursing. Each has been awarded a three-year scholarship to the school. The future nurses are Linda M. McCrory, 17, Clarissa B. Flippin, 18, and Jacqueline M. Gladney, 18, all students at McClymonds High and Clarice Ilean Brooks, 19, of Castlemont High. The winners were selected by counselors in the Oakland public high schools.

He later described an afternoon in 1970 when he'd been walking in that neighborhood along Piedmont Avenue and saw a possibility to follow his ambition: "I saw the Kaiser school. I walked in and talked to Josephine Coppedge. She told me she had been an Army nurse anesthetist. I asked her, 'Do you ever think of taking in any guys in this class?'" He was delighted with her answer, which, he reported, was "I'm going to be taking military people starting next year. I'll take five of them." His response was an immediate, "How do I sign up?"[27]

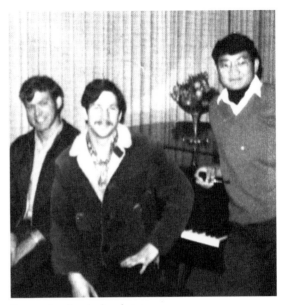

Encouraging diversity by admitting men.

True to her word, Coppedge and the faculty began admitting men in 1970. Purtle and four other men, all with medical military or police science experience, began nurses' training in the fall of 1971.

Having men in the school had required a number of changes, according to Purtle: "The gals wore yellow smocks over white nurses' dresses.[28] I wore a white smock with buttons on the side going out towards the shoulder, and a pair of white pants with white tennis shoes."[29]

More important than the difference in their school uniforms was the fact that male students were unable to fully participate in student life. So much of student life revolved around the dormitory, but there wasn't room for men there, so they had to live off campus. The men could take advantage of the extensive school library on the third floor for research and study, but they had to leave the dormitory building by 10 o'clock each night, making it hard to form study groups with their female classmates (these often went late into the night). At that time, decades before co-ed dormitories, it also meant male students missed participating in many of the informal extracurricular activities centered in the residence that helped their female classmates to bond.

Faculty member Bea Rudney saw a great deal that was positive in the changing makeup of the student body: "For the first time, we admitted male students and we were admitting older students, many of whom had degrees in other fields. They didn't have to live in the dorm. It made a great difference. I think they were helpful to the younger ones. They had a broader world view than the 18-year-old students."[30]

While Purtle went on to graduate, he noted that the other four men in his class went a different route. According to Purtle, in their junior year, Coppedge arranged a meeting for the five male students with Oakland police recruiters. With military and police backgrounds and now nurse training, although incomplete, they had become excellent candidates for the Oakland Police Department. They were offered immediate employment as police officers at a very attractive salary. Purtle, whose goal still was to become a nurse anesthetist, was the only one who turned down the offer and went on to earn a KFSN diploma.[31]

Coppedge seemed determined to offer female students alternative careers if they were not sure they wanted to pursue a nursing career. She arranged a similar seminar with airline representatives for those who were considering becoming what then were called stewardesses, as airlines gave preference to RNs for employment at that time.

In addition to the men at KFSN, there already was another group of students who were living off campus — the married female students. Originally, marriage had been grounds for immediate dismissal — but from the beginning, there had been exceptions. Probably the first one had been Francine Weir Ammerman, class of '50, whose story was told in Chapter Two. Three months before graduation, her Marine fiancé had been ordered to Korea. Sixty-seven years later, sitting in her kitchen, Francine looked at her husband and, smiling at the recollection, said, "Dorothea gave us three days off and we were able to get married before he had to leave."[32]

Although the rule against student marriages remained in effect, there were more and more exceptions as time went on. When Clair Lisker was asked how the rule got changed, she explained, "Actually, it was the students who wanted the change. We also had recruited some married students. I don't think we ever formalized it, it just seemed to happen. We also let the married students live out of the dorm if they wanted. I know that in the '70s we had lots of married students."[33]

Faculty member Cynthia Reed recalls that for the students, "Living in the residence was a real bonding experience. When the going got tough, they would have a built-in support system."[34] On the other hand, not having such easy access to the support of their classmates made school a little more difficult for male students and the married young women.

It was actually her marriage that brought Mary Ann Healy Thode, class of '66, to KFSN. She already had finished her first year at Providence Hospital's nursing school. "I had to leave Providence when I got married," she said, "because at that point, Catholic nursing schools didn't allow students to be married, so I transferred to Kaiser."[35]

Having married students led to some unexpected problems for Coppedge, but she solved them with imagination and grace. Lesley Meriwether, class of '63, had married in her junior year, moved into a

---
Having married students led to some unexpected problems for Coppedge, but she solved them with imagination and grace.

---

nearby apartment with her new husband and was expecting a baby in her final year of school. As class president, she was to give a speech at graduation. The problem was that she was in an advanced stage of pregnancy and the regular school uniform would have looked awkward and unflattering.

"When it came time for me to give the graduating speech, there was a lot of conflict between Mrs. Coppedge and myself about whether or not I should wear a girdle," Meriwether recalled. "I needed to be able to wear a uniform. She ended up ordering uniforms with a loose front that everyone wore so that I could participate, [and give] the graduating speech. I was so appreciative about that."[36]

The director and the faculty were anxious that the married women living off campus with their husbands have as much opportunity as possible to bond and develop friendships and support

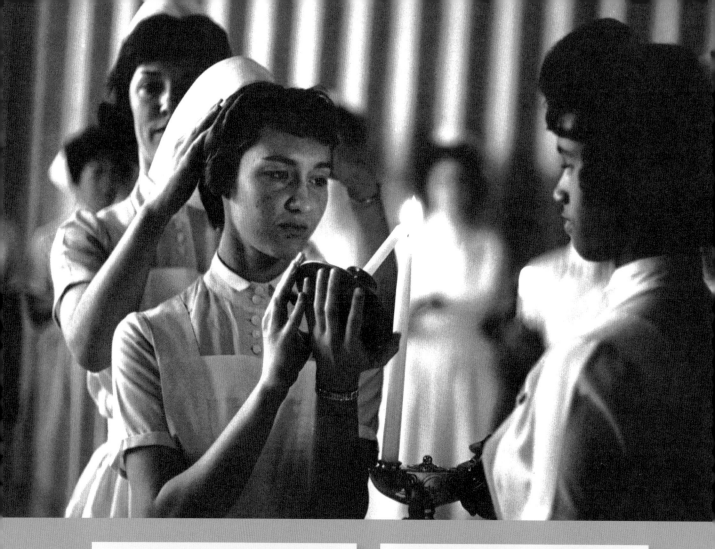

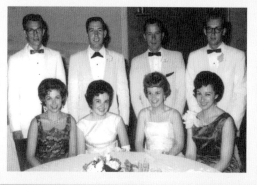

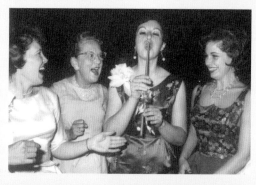

(Top to bottom) At Capping Ceremony, Freshman
receives her cap while Senior passes flame from her candle.

Candle-passing at formal dance – Claremont Hotel
Berkeley, California.

among their classmates who were living in the dorm. That was why, even though they had an apartment with their husbands, they were assigned a dormitory room, so they could study late with their friends and participate in the informal activities of their classmates. Thode was one of those married students with a dormitory room; she recalled that "you had to pay the same amount whether you were married or not, so you could stay there if you wanted. I had a roommate for both years."[37]

STUDENT TRADITIONS: CANDLE PASSING

By the 1960s a new tradition had taken root. It was called "candle passing," and it was a way of announcing an engagement for the whole class to celebrate.

When a student became engaged, she would tell one person, usually her best friend, that she would like to have a candle passing. Soon an anonymous note would be posted on the bulletin board, "Candle passing at 5:30 p.m." This would set off a flurry of excited speculations about who was going to be announcing her engagement that evening.

The ceremony usually took place on the dormitory's upper floor in a community room with the lights turned low for atmosphere. The centerpiece of the ritual was a candle set into an arrangement that resembled a wedding bouquet. The engagement ring was attached to the candle that then was lit.

Janice Price Klein, class of '63, who would marry a California Maritime Academy cadet she'd met at one of the many KFSN/CMA dances, described the joyful rituals: "They usually took place with everybody sitting on the floor in the dorm. The candle passing involved unmarried instructors and unmarried student nurses. You'd give your ring to whomever you had arranging this and she would tie your ring on the candle. We would sit on the floor in a circle and the candle would be passed around."[38]

Some girls would pretend they were the bride-to-be, sing some romantic songs that were popular at the time and they would start to blow out the candle. Then they would laugh, "No, I was just kidding!" and the candle would continue hand to hand around the circle, three times. Finally, the recently engaged student would end the suspense by blowing the candle out. They would offer congratulations, best wishes, hugs and then more laughter followed as the classmates celebrated together.

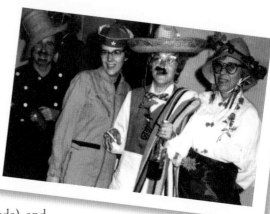

According to Jo Michael Beard Duke, class of '73, in her time "Candle passings were very common because a lot of the girls would go to dances at the base (Naval Air Station Alameda), and there was always somebody engaged every week, unengaged and engaged again!"[39]

A TIME OF NATIONAL SOCIAL TURMOIL

While the '60s were a time of great social upheaval around civil rights, with some exceptions, graduates don't remember it touching campus life — perhaps they were so immersed in the challenges of their academic and clinical studies, and perhaps because the school already was an example of a successful diverse community. Helen Harrison Robinson, one of the African American students, participated in a sit-in demonstration at a local restaurant's lunch counter. She felt it was something that she needed to do. "Some of the students saw me sitting there. 'There's Helen!' I said, 'I'll be right there as soon as I finish.'" When asked whether there had been any pushback from the school, she answered, "No, not that I know of. If there was, it wasn't enough to stop me from graduating."[40]

Students, however, did come face to face with the Vietnam War during their psychiatric clinical rotation at the VA Hospital in Martinez. There they saw firsthand the toll the war was taking on the young soldiers who'd been sent to Southeast Asia. The young women brought with them compassion, companionship and entertainment. The June 1967 KP Reporter described the "Spring Sing," when each of the three classes performed original musical skits for the veterans.

GRADUATION AND TAKING THE STATE BOARDS

The climax of three years at KFSN was the graduation ceremony. During the previous years, the school had celebrated the time-honored traditions of the nursing profession, including the capping ceremony, and the pinning ceremony, with candle lighting and the Nightingale Pledge. The nursing school also had developed its own graduation traditions. One that brings wide smiles to the faces of the alumni when they gather at school reunions is the chance to sing the school song (sung to the traditional graduation tune "Pomp and Circumstance"):

Here's to Kaiser Foundation,
Friend kind and true.
Tried through the ages,
Soul of honor are you.
We as nurses uphold you,
Bear your standards on high.
We rally to guide you,
Shout your praises to the sky;
Friend of our youth, God bless you,
Keep you as years go by.

The graduation ceremonies were formal affairs consisting of two services: a baccalaureate service followed by a graduation service. Students outfitted in their graduation uniforms initially filed down the aisle of the First Plymouth Congregational Church for a special baccalaureate service and later the First Presbyterian Church for the graduation ceremony. An audience of family and loved ones watched proudly as the men and women graduating — the women carrying a small bouquet of flowers, a gift from the school — walked across a flower-bedecked stage to receive their diploma and school pin from the hand of the director. Speakers included Kaiser Foundation Board of Trustees members and Kaiser Permanente executives, the director and some of the most outstanding students in the graduating class, such as the class president.

The first graduation speech had been delivered by Henry J. Kaiser himself — a statement of the importance of the school of nursing to him and his wife, Bess. Kaiser deeply held a conviction that there was no profession more compassionate or noble than that of a nurse.

Once a student had received her (or his) KFSN diploma, the final hurdle was the standardized examination all nursing school graduates must pass to become registered nurses licensed to practice in California. This examination was administered by the State Board of Nurse Examiners, today known as the California Board of Registered Nursing. Its mission was, and continues to be, to "protect and advocate for the health and safety of the public by ensuring the highest quality registered nurses in the State of California."[41]

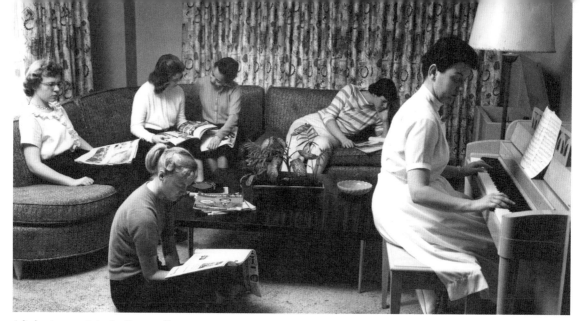

A little piano music in the Common Room.

Because the examinations are standardized and each applicant is given an identical test, they are one way of judging the effectiveness of the training received in each of California's schools of nursing. Coppedge and the faculty had set out to make KFSN the finest nursing school in California, and these tests helped judge their progress. Each year, the results had been increasingly gratifying. Each year, the faculty had made improvements in the curriculum, and each year, the scores rose.

The faculty may have known their students were well-prepared to take the state boards. Understandably though, students with so much riding on their test results weren't as confident, and spent many anxious days getting ready. They felt even more pressure knowing they not only were taking the test for themselves, they were representing KFSN. Some faculty told the students the same sentences that have been passed on from teachers to students for generations: "There is no use cramming at this late date. If you don't know it now, you never will." Even with such well-meaning assurances, many students wanted to "bone up" for the coming exam.

One instructor who offered to help was Clair Lisker. Nelle Neighbor Alonzo, class of '71, was one of the many very appreciative students who took advantage of Lisker's offer: "Clair Lisker was wonderful. She'd get all us young women together at her house for a study session. We'd go over things that would be pertinent for the test."[42]

Typically, KFSN students entered the examination room nervous but well prepared. After the tests, many told of gathering with classmates outside in the lobby, "What's wrong, why are we finished and the others are still there?"

Jeff Purtle was one of the KFSN students who was surprised at how well prepared they had been for the boards. "It took almost a full day to take the boards. It was in three sections. I thought, 'I can't be the first one done, there's something wrong,' so I went over everything again and I still was the first one done."[43] Students were so well prepared for their boards that for the first 18 years not a single KFSN student failed the examination.

The faculty paid close attention to the results of the boards, in particular to the scores in their specialty. Marion Yeaw, who joined the faculty in 1953, remembers the results of the state boards with pride. When she first arrived at the school,

———— • ————

Students were so well prepared for their boards that for the first 18 years not a single KFSN student failed the examination.

————————

the test results had been, in her words, "very respectable." However, after MacLean took over the scores went up each year. Yeaw was quick to add she thought this was not due to any failing of Dorothea Daniels who, in addition to putting a new faculty in place, had also been responsible for running the Nursing Department at the Oakland Hospital. She was stretched thin. Yeaw pointed out that it takes time to develop a faculty and curriculum.

Under the direction of Coppedge, spurred on by the faculty, the curriculum continued to improve as the faculty expanded and shared experience and ideas. It paid off. KFSN consistently scored in the top three of all the schools of nursing in the state, as described in Chapter 3.

The difference in KFSN patient-centered training began to show long before graduation and state boards. When students' rotations took them to non-Kaiser hospitals to continue their education alongside students from other nursing schools in the Bay Area, the supervising physicians and nursing staff of those facilities saw a higher level of patient and clinical experience in the KFSN-trained nurses. Juliette Whitfield Powell, class of '58, realized there was something special about

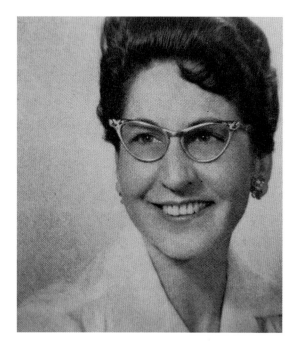

The phrase, "They know how to take care of patients" was a direct reflection of the success the school was having with patient-centered medicine. The school's philosophy and the efforts of the administration and faculty to implement it were paying off in the near term — and reimagining the future of nursing education and the delivery of caring for patients in the Kaiser Permanente way that continues to this day. ◉

———— • ————

"They know how to take care of patients."

————————

her education during her communicable disease rotation at what today is known as San Francisco General Hospital.

"It was called City and County then," Powell recalled. "Mount Zion, UC San Francisco, Kaiser and a couple of other schools rotated their students there, two or three students from each school, only two from our school. It was a scary place. Most of the patients we were dealing with [had] TB. The instructor who assigned the patients would say, 'We'll give this patient to a UC student, no, wait a moment, we'll give her to a Kaiser nurse, they know how to take care of patients.'"[44]

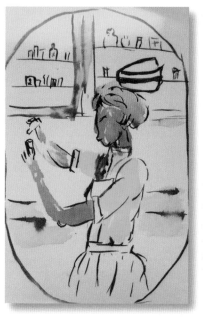

(Top left to bottom)
Mrs. Coppedge.

Student's creativity.

(Opposite) Student nurse scrubbing for surgery during OR rotation, c. 1962.

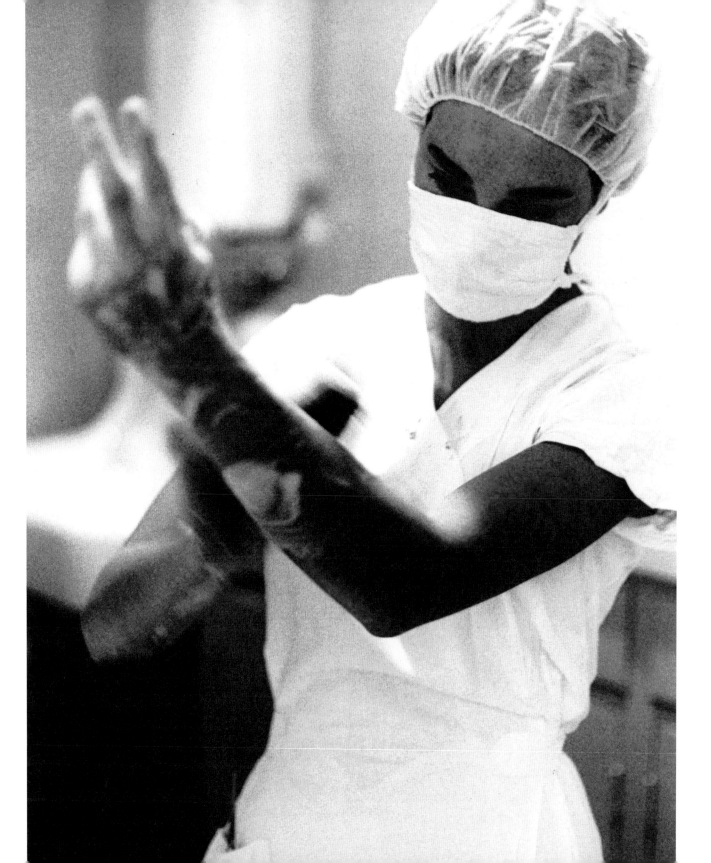

Graduation class ready to embark on their nursing careers.

CLOSING of KFSN

A LEADER IN NURSING EDUCATION 5 LAUNCHES A LIVING LEGACY

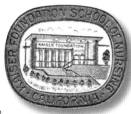

NATIONAL NURSING ORGANIZATIONS CALL FOR A CHANGE IN NURSING EDUCATION. The 1960s and '70s were an exciting time in clinical medicine. Coronary bypass surgery was saving hundreds and then thousands of lives, and ICUs were becoming increasingly effective in the care of seriously ill patients. Limb reattachments were no longer front-page news, made possible by the development of powerful immunosuppressant drugs, and successful liver, lung and heart transplant operations were becoming increasingly common in leading hospitals across the country.

Accelerated medical progress and supporting technologies already had placed new demands on nurses and the schools that were preparing students for practice in the '70s, '80s and beyond. Since 1960, nursing education had undergone major changes. Schools offering a variety of nursing programs took anywhere from two to five years to complete, and led to varying levels of nursing responsibilities.

Leaders in the nursing profession and, in particular, the National League for Nursing (NLN), were pushing to reduce this to just two levels of nursing education: the two-year associate degree and the four-year baccalaureate degree. The American Nurses Association was calling for a baccalaureate degree as entry into practice. Graduates of three-year diploma schools already were starting to face discrimination in hiring and promotion. It was apparent that KFSN was facing an uncertain future unless it could adapt to the new conditions and expectations within the profession.

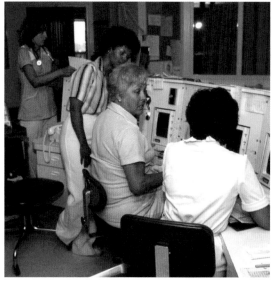
ICU console c. 1964.

———— • ————

This completely nontraditional approach to nursing education, where clinical rotations were limited strictly to experiential learning, had been the guiding educational philosophy from the early days of the school, and the results had transformed it into one of the nation's leading nursing schools.

As part of a search for ways to improve the KFSN curriculum and meet the new challenges, Director Josephine Coppedge and Helen Ross, the school's chief operating officer, attended a convention of the NLN in Denver in 1965, where they heard a presentation on a proposed radical change in nursing education.

Until this time, the key feature of the KFSN curriculum, refined over the years, had been the careful integration of classroom theory with clinical practice. There was a reciprocal reinforcement of classroom learning and immediate and related clinical experience. This completely nontraditional approach to nursing education, where clinical rotations were limited strictly to experiential learning, had been the guiding educational philosophy from the early days of the school, and the results had transformed it into one of the nation's leading nursing schools. However, the presentation in Denver proposed curriculum changes that would turn education at KFSN upside down.

Upon their return from the NLN convention, Coppedge and Ross designed a proposed change in the KFSN curriculum. Under the Coppedge-Ross plan, faculty would teach students in the clinical divisions – pediatrics, obstetrics and gynecology, psychiatry, medical/surgical nursing, operating room, emergency room and home health – by looking at nursing care in each division from a birth to death perspective rather than a specialty perspective. This was a major change, and to a faculty used to developing curricula and fine tuning it themselves, this total rearrangement of the curriculum came as an unwelcome shock.

No longer would there be that close coordination between classroom and clinical. It didn't matter what department the students were rotating through. For example, students on a surgical rotation would have information presented to them in terms of issues at different stages of the patients' lives rather than the theory of caring for surgical patients. Students would not have the theoretical knowledge they needed to understand what they were seeing clinically. However, the approach had sounded promising to Coppedge and Ross. On the train returning to Oakland from Denver, the two women had laid out how they would present the new approach to the faculty. It was not an easy sell.

Over the years, particularly since 1953 when the school had become independent from the

hospital, KFSN faculty had taken a guiding role in the development of the curriculum. Changes had been made by consensus, and the result had been a curriculum that was both innovative and effective. Now they were being told to accept these sudden and major changes to a curriculum that had evolved over a decade and had been proven effective.

Faculty members were taken aback by the suggestion that they upend an educational process that was providing outstanding results in favor of the Denver curriculum. However, they did not go into open revolt. Although she and the faculty were opposed to the changes, Curriculum Coordinator Clair Lisker and the faculty made a good faith effort to integrate the new principles based on the "From Life to Death" approach.

"We tried to see where we could integrate it, and I think may actually [have] had advantages in getting people to think differently and to ask themselves, 'Why are we doing this? Can we somehow look at it more broadly, and where can we teach that more broadly and then integrate it into the clinical divisions?'" Lisker said. "We compromised. We decided that we would try to incorporate these principles into the theory that was being taught, so that they could function safely in their clinical divisions. It was a constant topic in faculty meetings. It really never worked out, so what happened was after six or maybe nine months we transitioned back into what we had been doing, theory and practice coordinated."[1]

To the relief of the faculty, the conflict in educational approach seemed to have had minimal effect on student scores on the state boards, as they continued to be among the highest of California's schools of nursing.[2]

IN SEARCH OF AN ACADEMIC PARTNER

While things may have settled down at the school by returning to the proven effective curriculum, the underlying issues remained. Advances in medicine meant nurses were being asked to take more and more responsibility. Nursing educators and their professional organizations were convinced that three-year schools were not turning out nurses prepared for the challenges of the 1970s and beyond.

KFSN already had recognized the need for advanced education in 1967, when it had become the first nursing school in California to offer an associate degree in addition to its RN diploma. As a result, graduates not only were well-prepared by the correlated curriculum, the seamless blending of theory and clinical experience, they were prepared to continue their education in nursing specialties after graduation.

Josephine Coppedge and the KFSN administration realized that more changes were needed. If the school was to retain its position as a leader in nursing education, its leaders might be forced to transform the school into a four-year baccalaureate program. They could not do this on their own; they would need to affiliate with a baccalaureate degree-granting college or university. They began looking for such a school.

Over a four-year period, St. Mary's College, College of the Holy Names, California State University Hayward, UC Berkeley and Golden Gate University were approached. Consultants were brought in to help with the transition, including Dr. Harkin Jones, who was on the faculty at UC Berkeley, and Dorothy Ozimek from the NLN.

A satisfactory education partner needed to meet several requirements. KFSN's partner would need to emphasize community-based medicine, prevention and the continuum of care. These became major sticking points with each of the schools that were approached as they, along with the accrediting body NLN, were unwilling to let clinical considerations determine academic syllabi, stating that curriculum design belonged to academia, not community partners. Further, they required that nursing degrees would be attributable to the name of the school of nursing associated with the degree-granting organization. This proved to be a major stumbling block.

Since the Kaiser Foundation would be providing funds for the program, the board of trustees wanted the Kaiser name attached to the program and wanted its students taught curriculum that represented Kaiser Permanente's fundamental values. Again, KFSN was ahead of its time, as names of funding organizations now are associated with schools, such as the Betty Irene Moore School of Nursing at UC Davis or The Valley Foundation School of Nursing at San Jose State University. Similarly, today's schools of nursing are calling upon clinical partners for input into curriculum to keep it relevant to the evolving health care delivery system.

During this time, the faculty was aware of this search for a suitable academic partner, but most believed it would be only a matter of time before a satisfactory arrangement would be made and KFSN would prepare for the possibility of becoming a four-year school.

Faculty members looked to other schools for ideas on how they might adapt KFSN's three-year curriculum to a four-year program. Cynthia Reed, OB instructor, thought a baccalaureate program might offer the opportunity to provide even more experience than was currently possible in the three-year program.[3]

It was not to be.

CLOSING OF THE SCHOOL

Since 1953, KFSN had been operating as a part of the Kaiser Foundation Health Plan, which was led by Clifford Keene, MD, as president. Keene reported to the Health Plan Board of Trustees, which also acted as the board of trustees of the nursing school. Now the board had directed Keene to prepare a report on the future of the school, bringing the board up to date on the search for an appropriate affiliation and to provide suggestions on how the school should proceed.

On Nov. 14, 1973, at a meeting of the school's board of trustees, Keene read his report aloud. He began by outlining changes taking place in the nursing profession, including the pressures to have only two basic nursing degrees, a two-year associate degree and a four-year baccalaureate degree. He described how this was causing a great many of the freestanding, hospital-based nursing schools similar to KFSN to close. He reported on the unsuccessful efforts of the school's management to develop a joint program with a university or college that would have made it possible for students to graduate in four years with a baccalaureate degree while still retaining their identity as Kaiser students.

He went on to say they also had investigated the possibility of KFSN itself becoming a degree-granting institution, and had concluded the obstacles to achieve academic accreditation were insurmountable. His conclusion was that it was no longer sensible for the foundation to operate the school, and recommended it be closed. His conclusion was put into the form of a motion:

"... No new students will be accepted by the school and that the school's educational program will be terminated in June, 1976, when the present Freshman class graduates; and that management is directed to take all steps necessary in order to assure maintenance of the school's educational standards and the quality of instruction between now and June, 1976."[4]

The motion was put to a vote and approved unanimously. After 25 years of innovation and excellence in training nurses, the days of the Kaiser Foundation School of Nursing now were numbered.

Several days later, the news that the school would be closing was announced to the students, who had assembled that morning in the Piedmont building to begin what they had expected to be a normal day. The stunning announcement caused a great deal of consternation, severe disappointment and even anger among the students, who immediately began wondering what this would mean for them. Would the seniors get to finish the year? What would happen to the juniors and to the freshmen who were just beginning their nursing education? Would they get a full nursing education with the same high standards the earlier classes had received?

The school administration had expected this reaction and had prepared for it. The entire student body — the classes of '74, '75 and '76 — was ushered onto buses already waiting in the school's parking lot. They were driven two miles across town to the main auditorium in the Kaiser Industries Headquarters building on Lake Merritt, where the surprised and upset students were told they would be given details about how the school's closing would affect them.

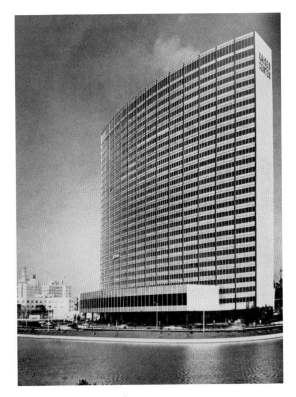

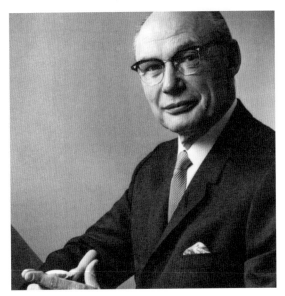

(Top to bottom) Kaiser Center, Kaiser Industries International Headquarters.

Clifford Keene, MD.

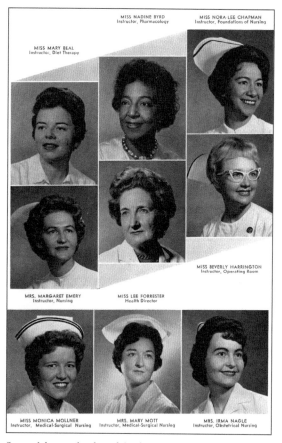

MISS NADINE BYRD
Instructor, Pharmacology

MISS NORA-LEE CHAPMAN
Instructor, Foundations of Nursing

MISS MARY BEAL
Instructor, Diet Therapy

MISS BEVERLY HARRINGTON
Instructor, Operating Room

MRS. MARGARET EMERY
Instructor, Nursing

MISS LEE FORRESTER
Health Director

MISS MONICA MOLLNER
Instructor, Medical-Surgical Nursing

MRS. MARY MOTT
Instructor, Medical-Surgical Nursing

MRS. IRMA NAGLE
Instructor, Obstetrical Nursing

Some of the greatly-admired faculty,
1963 Yearbook.

The mood in the auditorium was somber, but what the students heard was reassuring. Although no new classes would enter the school, the present students would all have the chance to graduate. They were told that KFSN had made a commitment to each of them and now promised to keep that commitment without compromising the quality of the training they would receive.

Even as the school moved nearer to its final closing date in June 1976, the quality of the students' classes and clinical experience remained high. For those members of the class of '76, there was an added pressure to succeed. Previously, if students had wanted to pause their program for some reason, perhaps to decide whether she or he wanted to continue nursing education or because of financial reasons, this could be done knowing they could return and join a later class. But after the announcement in November 1973, there would not be a later class.

Some school traditions necessarily fell by the wayside. One was the Big Sister–Little Sister relationship that had been the beginning of scores of life-long friendships. It couldn't continue since there weren't going to be any more students starting at the school. Another tradition that disappeared was the school yearbook. The rationale is not clear, but the class of 1974, which was the last class to graduate from a "full" school with three classes, was also the last class to have a yearbook.

To instructor Bea Rudney, without a full student body, the school felt like a skeleton of its former self. Some faculty, those whose teaching assignments had been primarily in the freshman class, also left. The Health Plan showed its appreciation by offering them jobs within the Health Plan or a generous separation payout. How they were treated offered reassurance to the remaining faculty that they, too, would be well treated when it was their time to leave, so there was surprisingly little turnover in the faculty for the remaining two years. This was one reason why the quality of the training remained high through the school's final days.

There was another reason Bea Rudney and others thought the school seemed strangely empty even though the last two classes were the largest in the school's history. Many students were living off campus. The makeup of the student body was changing. These last classes contained more married students, they were older than the other students, and some of them were mothers with young children. Their experience of the school was somewhat different than that of the students who while training lived in the old Piedmont Hotel. They lived off campus and not under the strict dormitory rules managing their comings and goings, study time and even how they dressed. When not on duty, they dressed far more casually than the dormitory dress code would allow. To the consternation of some faculty, the younger students started adopting this casual dress style, so the student body was even looking a bit different.

Some things didn't change. For instance, candle passings were still a part of dormitory life as girls celebrated their engagements. (With breakups and new engagements, some students had more than one!) Capping ceremonies and graduations continued to be held at the same Presbyterian church, only a few blocks from the hospital.

At her capping ceremony, Sharon Tolton Scolnick, class of '76, a single mother, was excited and proud to have reached this milestone and brought her two daughters, 3 and 6 years old, to the ceremony. To ensure their behavior, she promised them that if they behaved, they would all go for ice cream when the ceremony was over. Standing with her class in front of the church facing the assembled relatives and friends for this time-honored ritual, Scolnick noticed her 3-year-old was starting to act out. Embarrassed, she ducked down behind the other students and snuck off stage, out the back door, and back in through a door into the congregation to get to her girls and settle them down. Then, as unobtrusively

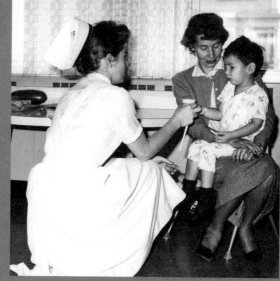
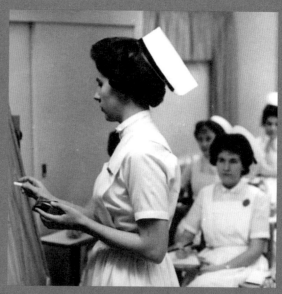
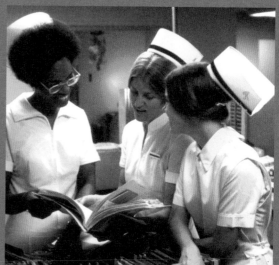
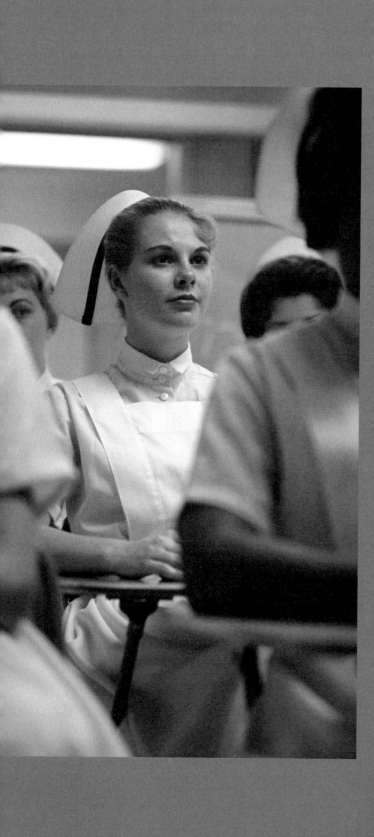

as possible, she returned through the side door and took her place among the proud students to receive her cap.[5]

Where a few years before, living off campus had meant those students lost the fellowship and support of their classmates, now there were enough day students that they could form their own study groups. They often had more in common with each other than they did with the younger students. As nonresident students, they could move about from one study group to another as they needed and as their family commitments allowed.

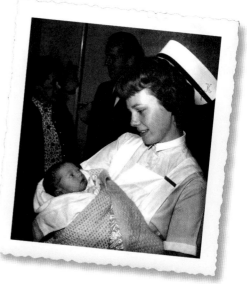

The study groups also were partly social, and they began having parties in some of their homes. Scolnick smiled as she remembered those groups: "We had some great study parties. There were probably two or three different groups and you could bounce in and out of the groups according to your study needs and your family obligations. You'd get together, have a glass of wine and start studying."[6]

Inevitably, the time of graduation came around for the class of 1976. On June 6, 1976, proud parents, relatives and friends gathered at the First Presbyterian Church of Oakland for the 26th and final graduation from the Kaiser Foundation School of Nursing. Ironically, it was the largest graduating class in the school's 29-year history: 50 women and four men.

While relatives and friends took their seats in the pews inside the church, the graduating students formed into orderly lines, shortest to the tallest, before entering and marching in to the front of the flower-bedecked church. Peter Guzman's strongest memory of that day is the powerful smell of the dozens of

(Opposite left) Student attentively listening to the lecture.

(Top to bottom) Student with mother and child on a home visit.

Students had the opportunity to lead in the classroom.

Student reviewing patient charts.

rose bouquets that decorated the church. Then the line of students returned to the seats prepared for them in the back of the church, where they waited for the beginning of the ceremonies.

For the last time as a class, the graduates sang the school song and recited the Nightingale Pledge. Then, one by one, as a name was called, that graduating student walked back down the aisle and crossed the same stage that every newly minted nurse had traversed since the school's first graduation in 1950. It was the same stage from which Henry Kaiser more than a quarter-century earlier had told the charter class, "It is my conviction that the careers of giving and serving which you have dedicated your lives to will give you true happiness — the most genuine kind of success and happiness there is on this earth."

When Claudia Walker Heinemann, the 1,065th graduate, crossed the stage to receive her diploma, the Kaiser Foundation School of Nursing had reached its end. However, inside the hearts and minds of those 1,065 graduates, the school was leaving a legacy that had been basic to a Kaiser Foundation School of Nursing diploma: an appreciation of the importance of community-based health care; a commitment to continuity of care; the value of preventive care; the importance of educating the patient and family; and of the need for active patient involvement in his or her own medical care. Wherever they went, graduates brought with them values fostered at KFSN for the benefit of their patients, for the organizations in which they would work, and for the nursing profession.

"The school certainly had an impact," said Jim Vohs, retired president and CEO of the Kaiser Foundation Health Plan. "Personally, I hated to see it close. I thought we were producing the best nurses in the state." Vohs went on to say, "it was the hardest job I had to do as president."[7]

John Smillie, MD, wrote in his excellent history of The Permanente Medical Group, "The school was an experiment that had run its course, but it had also enriched the Permanente philosophy with a sympathy and respect for the nursing profession as an essential component of group practice medicine."[8]

This would not have come as a surprise to Naomi Eiko Tanikawa, class of '54A, who almost a quarter-century before had written in the school newspaper, The Drawsheet: "We believe the day

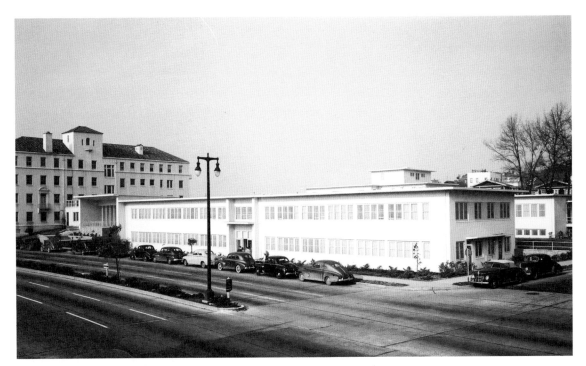

Oakland Hospital, c. early 1950s.

will come when KFSN will be recognized as one of the leaders in progressive nursing education."

The Kaiser Foundation School of Nursing began addressing problems and obstacles with courageous leadership, a bold passion for pragmatic efficiency even when it defied the status quo, and a relentless pursuit of excellence and innovation across a continuum of care. Innovative concepts emerged most notably in the areas of leadership, culture, diversity and curriculum. KFSN and Kaiser Permanente challenged the sick care model, reshaped the delivery of nursing education and elevated nursing's professional practice. This legacy of disruptive innovation is integral to the structure and culture of Kaiser Permanente and its commitment to professional nursing practice today.

Nurse Scholars Academy
graduating class 2019.

EPILOGUE

THE LEGACY 6 CONTINUES

KFSN GRADUATES SHAPED THE FUTURE OF NURSING: AN ONGOING EXPRESSION OF ITS LEGACY. Since the school's closing in 1976, KFSN graduates have made their mark in many venues, reaching far into all aspects of health care and beyond. Their high-caliber, innovative education was evident in all aspects of their work. Graduates were held in very high esteem, and set the standard of what hospital administrators and physicians expected from all nurses.

They promoted and practiced the underlying values of the Kaiser Permanente way of providing health care — all with a great deal of pride as part of the Kaiser family and its dedication to health plan members and the community. Through their practice, Kaiser graduates helped shape the care delivery system Kaiser Permanente continues to follow today.

KFSN graduates were exemplary staff nurses — leading the way in providing the best patient care, whether at the hospital bedside, in the clinic, at home or in the community. They became advance practice nurses, nurse managers and administrators, high-ranking health care executives, physicians, educators and professors, psychotherapists and behavior health specialists. They became authors, missionaries, innovators in the delivery of health care, lawyers, entrepreneurs, policy makers and even politicians.[1]

Some graduates furthered their education and joined the ranks of California's first nurse practitioners. Many followed the expectation of continuing their education by obtaining professional certification, baccalaureate, master's and doctoral degrees. An overwhelming number of graduates worked at Kaiser Permanente facilities — some for a few years and some for their entire professional career — committed to the philosophy of health care that was embedded in their education.

Upon the school's closing, the alumni were honored by Kaiser Permanente's board and executive leadership with these words: " ... the School's last class will graduate tomorrow. The School's name and reputation, however, will be perpetuated by its honor roll of graduate registered nurses as they continue their service to others."[2]

CONTINUING THE LEGACY THROUGH INNOVATION IN NURSING PRACTICE
NURSE PRACTITIONERS

Kaiser Permanente's use of nurse practitioners (NP) dates back to 1965, when the concept of NPs began through the leadership of Loretta Ford, RN, Ed.D., and Henry Silver, MD, at the University of Colorado. The role was first established in pediatrics.

When Dr. Sidney Garfield heard about this newly defined use of registered nurses with advanced training, he dispatched Dr. Clifford Keene, then vice president and general manager of Kaiser Foundation Hospital, the Kaiser Foundation Health Plan and KFSN, to Colorado to learn more about it. It seemed like an effective way to meet the physician shortage and have these specially trained nurses care for well children, freeing up the doctors to care for ill children who needed a higher level of medical care.

Soon thereafter, NPs were introduced to Kaiser Permanente through The Permanente Medical Group (TPMG) physicians in Oakland, California, first under the leadership of Dr. Ed Schoen, a pediatrician, and then later Dr. Steve Taller in adult medicine. At that time, there were no programs available to train these advance practice nurses in California, so the medical group began its own training program.

Southern California Permanente Medical Group (SCPMG) soon followed suit, using nurses in specialty and extended roles in pediatrics, but without the title of NP. In 1964, SCPMG had hired its first nurse to provide well baby care, working in partnership and under the supervision of a pediatrician.[3] This was a precursor to the NP movement that began at the University of Colorado.

TPMG physicians consulted with Clair Lisker, who was curriculum coordinator at KFSN at the time, to determine whether KFSN graduates had the ability and training to adapt to this role. The University of Colorado's NP program faculty brought their program to Oakland to help TPMG set up its program. Lisker advised on curriculum and teaching design to facilitate KFSN graduates' transition into the role. Because nurse practitioners' training was supervised by Permanente physicians, they were easily integrated into the medical care staff.

Not knowing how to classify NPs, the decision was made to take the staff nurse classification under the California Nurses Association (CNA) labor agreement and add a salary increase to it, since the nurses trained by TPMG came from the staff nurse ranks. Thus, from the beginning, the NPs in northern California were part of CNA, setting a precedent within Kaiser Permanente.

TPMG trained Phyllis Plant Moroney, class of '57A, as its first nurse practitioner in a formal program in 1968. Moroney described her pediatric nurse practitioner training thusly: "We weren't trained in sick children care; we were trained in well child behavior and care. We specialized in talking to moms about day-to-day things, but we did see ear infections [and] sore throats."[4]

Besides conducting examinations, patient education was an important part of an NP's responsibilities. Patient education in a pediatric setting was a natural extension of KFSN graduates' training, which included patient and family education, making this an easy addition to their NP practice. Moroney added, "We did a lot of teaching. That's one thing that physicians aren't trained to do. They aren't trained in teething, breast feeding, toilet training and sibling rivalry. However, we were also taught sick child care, to the point that we recognized when something was abnormal and then referred the child to the pediatrician."[5]

Early on, Kaiser Permanente also hired NPs who were trained elsewhere, such as at the University of Colorado, but archives indicate that Moroney was the first NP trained in California.

Health plan members liked the NPs. Moroney remembers how she used to remind the patients, "I am a nurse practitioner, I am not a doctor, and they would answer, 'I know, doctor, but ... you're the best person I've had to take care of me (or my children). I feel so comfortable with you.'"[6]

SCPMG concurrently expanded its early use of clinical nurse specialists who worked in tandem with pediatricians into what would be SCPMG's formal program to train NPs in pediatrics, internal medicine and OB/GYN. SCPMG launched this training program in 1971.

While Kaiser wasn't the first health system to use NPs and KFSN graduates were not the first nurse practitioners, Kaiser Permanente's NPs had a great impact on the acceptance of NPs as providers in the nation's health care systems. The concept of NPs spread in part because of Kaiser Permanente's experiences with them. Once again, Kaiser Permanente was in the forefront of innovative care delivery. Graduates of its school of nursing were beginning to create a KFSN legacy through their innovative practice, firmly cementing the value of NPs in our nation's health care delivery system.

As colleges and universities began developing NP programs, the California Board of Registered Nursing (BRN) assumed jurisdiction over NP practice. In 1980, the BRN called for voluntary certification of NPs, followed by mandatory certification in 1984.[7] The NP programs provided by both TPMG and SCPMG officially were recognized in 1980, giving them the full status that NPs completing college-based programs received.[8] In 1975, SCPMG's program had become affiliated with the California State University Los Angeles School of Nursing, offering continuing education and a certificate with SCPMG staff training the NPs.[9] TPMG training of NPs was discontinued in 1977, as colleges and universities took over the preparation of NPs.

NURSE-MANAGED MULTIPHASIC HEALTH ASSESSMENT PROGRAM

About two years after the pediatric NP program was established, its success had a major impact in another area of medical practice, the multiphasic program. Multiphasic was an innovative idea of Drs. Morris Collen and Sidney Garfield. It was a highly organized, semi-computerized screening program designed to improve the efficiency of an overloaded medical care system by having members go through a complete initial health assessment. It separated members into three major groups: the well, the worried well and the sick.[10]

Garfield soon realized the semi-automated multiphasic physical examination could be carried out by nonphysicians (called paraprofessionals by Garfield). At first Garfield thought they could be run by nurses who had been trained to work in the multiphasic clinic. When he learned there were no nurses who knew how to do physical examinations or health evaluations, and furthermore, there were no training programs to prepare them to do it, Garfield's reaction was, "find good nurses and train them."[11]

A search began to find TPMG physicians who were willing to take on this multifaceted project while simultaneously designing a new training program for medical nurse practitioners. Six nurses were selected and trained simultaneously to be NPs and set up an organized health evaluation and triage unit. KFSN graduate La Verne Oyarzo, class of '54, helped organize the program and became one of its first NPs. She was the nurse leader of the program as well as a student. The NPs were a major success, and their responsibili-

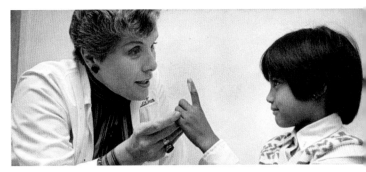

Phyllis Plant Moroney, KP's first trained NP.

ties grew as they proved their value by improving access and delivering high-quality care. Soon, their practice extended into obstetrics and later into adult medicine.

FAMILY-CENTERED PERINATAL CARE PROGRAM

Another example of nurse-led innovation in care delivery was FAMCP, the Family-Centered Perinatal Care Program.[12] It was developed by KFSN graduate Deloras Plake Jones, class of '63.

Jones, along with her physician colleagues — neonatologist Dr. Mark Yanover and obstetrician Dr. Michael Miller — designed and implemented a nurse-run model of care for low-risk obstetrical patients and their newborns.

This innovative approach to maternity care was designed as a response to a societal change that was occurring among young parents. It was offered as an alternative to home deliveries, which were becoming increasing popular in the late 1960s and early 1970s for young families that did not want traditional hospital-based maternity care.

Many young parents thought hospital births were too impersonal and did not meet the needs of those who wanted a more natural and humanistic approach to the birthing experience. FAMCAP included preparing parents for early discharge and sending the family home as early as six hours after a hospital birth, with follow-up care given at home by nurse practitioners. FAMCAP was a forerunner and a model for early discharge programs for low-risk obstetrical patients that ultimately became the norm throughout the country, with most discharges occurring 24 hours after the birth.

Published evidence-based outcomes research that accompanied the program's development influenced the American College of Obstetrics and Gynecology and the American Academy of Pediatrics standards for early discharge of low-risk obstetrical patients.[13, 14, 15] This nurse-run program, developed by a KFSN graduate in partnership with physician colleagues, once again put Kaiser Permanente in the forefront of care delivery — another example of continuing the legacy of KFSN.

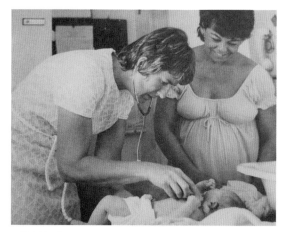

FAMCAP NP examines newborn at home while mom watches.

Alumnus in full uniform stands next to statue on dedication day, June 2015.

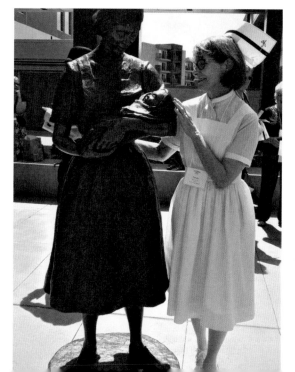

EXPANDED ROLE OF THE NURSE

A shortage of physicians and the growing needs of an expanding health plan member base generated a demand for more trained health care providers. As in the past, challenges created opportunities for innovation.

The organization once again looked to see how nurses could be utilized in different ways, building upon the positive experiences with nurse practitioners and the high quality of care and patient satisfaction their practice produced. From the mid-1980s through late 1990s, nurses demonstrated how they could contribute to patient care as well as to the health of their communities. It also demonstrated the innovative approach that was one of KFSN's legacy elements: Nurses trained in the "Permanente Way" of practicing prevention, promotion and wellness as central to total health.

The important role of the nurse practitioner became firmly established in caring for Kaiser Permanente health plan members. Furthermore, the use of NPs within Kaiser Permanente strengthened the importance of this growing role for nurses throughout the nation. During this time, Kaiser Permanente was the largest employer of NPs in California.

In the early 1990s, the physician shortage also opened the door for nurses to practice in extended roles. The Nurse Practice Act, through the California BRN, allowed registered nurses to legally extend their roles beyond the normal scope of practice of an RN under standardized procedures (SP).[16]

SPs are developed following specific criteria approved by participating nurses, physicians and the organization's administration. The extended role includes aspects of care usually carried out by a physician and provides for independently caring for patients within defined parameters and under the supervision of a physician. These roles or functions also could be filled by NPs and physician assistants (PAs).

Performing screening sigmoidoscopies, taking a patient's history in preparation for surgical procedures and serving as surgical first assistant are examples of how nurses functioned in extended roles. Another extended role was the newly designated position of case manager, who managed and coordinated the care of patients with chronic diseases, working in partnership with physicians who managed the acute or more critical aspects of their care. This role gave the nurse an extended scope of practice and authority with patients, which included managing the medications of patients with chronic diseases.

Nurse-run clinics also began during this time, with nurses managing wound clinics, travel clinics or well-baby clinics, as well as those for patients with such chronic diseases as diabetes or congestive heart failure, in which patient education was especially important.

Although nurses continue to practice in extended roles today, some roles have become mainstream nursing practice, albeit with additional education, such as care managers. Other roles, such as nurses doing screening sigmoidoscopies, were eliminated in the late 1990s as TPMG hired more physicians. Nevertheless, the groundwork was laid for appreciating the scope of care an RN could provide.

Advice nurses got their start at this time, with call centers operating 24 hours a day. Advice Nurse Manuals were required to facilitate manually looking up best-practice protocols, as this was before the availability of electronic databases. Early on, some of the advice nurses even took calls from their homes at night, before the volume required onsite centralized services to be open around the clock.

This practice of RNs giving real-time advice on the telephone is now a hallmark of Kaiser Permanente care. The organization was a leader in this practice, which developed about the same time as telemedicine. Telemedicine has become an important means of providing care, especially in remote areas and even where direct patient contact is needed, without the provider actually being on site.

CONTINUING THE LEGACY THROUGH NURSING EDUCATION

Joint ventures with academia provided Kaiser Permanente nurses access to higher education, following the legacy element and framework first established with KFSN when the school of nursing was established in 1947. Throughout the organization's history, access to higher education has been a priority; this continued into the 21st century with Kaiser Permanente's support and development of the California Collaborative Model for Nursing Education (CCMNE) in the early 2000s through the Kaiser Permanente Health Education Workforce Fund.[17]

As a result of this pioneering work, nearly all California community colleges are members of a collaborative with a baccalaureate-granting school of nursing, greatly improving access to a BSN education for associate degree-prepared nurses, thus leading to a more highly educated workforce in California.

The legacy of access to higher education was launched in 1988 under the leadership of the Northern California Region's chief nurse executive, Deloras Plake Jones, class of '63, when Kaiser Permanente developed a joint venture with the University of San Francisco (USF) to make baccalaureate education accessible to associate degree- or diploma-prepared staff nurses.[18] This innovative program was one of the first distance education programs in the country.

The newly established Nursing Teleconferencing Network, with Multimedia Department leader Bob Bodine serving as its champion, provided access to classes that were broadcast from the regional offices to six medical centers across the region. Nurses received the lectures in the evenings (after work) in a group-learning venue with facilitated discussions. USF, in its continuing innovative and flexible approach to nursing education, discounted the tuition, saving the students 60 percent. Forty associate degree and diploma-prepared KP nurses participated in that first 15-month program and received their BSN.

Debora Zachau, an associate degree-educated nurse who went on to become director of women's health and pediatrics, was a young nurse wondering how she ever would be able to obtain her bachelor's degree, as she was working full time and had children. Zachau recalls that KP gave her the opportunity she needed by offering the joint venture with USF in an evening program broadcast at a nearby Kaiser hospital.

"The opportunity to attend the joint venture program with USF was life changing," Zachau said. "It offered skills in nursing and leading teams. I was introduced to Kaiser senior leaders who were supporting the program. Their confidence... empowered myself and others. I feel the contributions I gave in my position(s) were so much due to this program. ... [as a result of this program], my career path changed. I was so pleased I took the journey I did and that Kaiser made it possible."[19]

In 1994, a joint venture was established with Sonoma State University through the distance education media that provided access to a master's degree in leadership or case management for Kaiser Permanente nurses. The format used in the USF/KP joint venture continued for graduate education.

Dorcas Walton, KP's regional director for nursing and clinical practice, recalls that she and her colleagues were novice nurse managers at the Santa Rosa Hospital, which they helped open. This new hospital began with shared governance and a professional practice that included differentiated practice roles. Even though Walton and the others only had a BSN, the expectation was set that they would get their master's degrees, as new nurse managers already were expected to have advanced degrees in their leadership roles. KP's arrangement with Sonoma State made that possible.

Walton noted that, "our advanced degrees set the standard for nurse managers in the community hospital and opened the door for me throughout my long career with Kaiser."[20]

The USF/KP demonstration program was duplicated into a more enduring model in a joint venture with Holy Names College in 1995. Clair O'Sullivan Lisker, class of '51A, upon her retirement from the Oakland hospital, along with Dr. Lois Welches, Kaiser Permanente's first nurse researcher, developed a very successful joint venture that reached out to nurses throughout the region. The program was extended to southern California in 1998 at 12 separate sites. Eventually, the program was transferred to California State University (CSU), Fullerton, enabling nurses outside of Kaiser Permanente to access a BSN education via the distance learning network — years before the advent of today's popular online education programs.

The fourth joint venture of note, demonstrating Kaiser Permanente's innovative approach to nursing education and further defining itself as a disruptive innovator to traditional care delivery, was the establishment of the certified registered nurse anesthetist (CRNA) program as a joint venture between TPMG and Samuel Merritt College (SMC) in 1994. Most of these CRNA graduates helped fill the void of anesthesiologists at Kaiser Permanente hospitals.

SCPMG had a long-established CRNA program in partnership with CSU Long Beach and then CSU Fullerton. The SCPMG and the SMC CRNA programs very creatively shared faculty through the Nursing Teleconferencing Network, once again setting Kaiser Permanente in the forefront of innovative approaches to nursing education. This innovative approach was a partnership between a private college and a state university, both with very different tuition and financial structures.

CONTINUING THE LEGACY THROUGH LEADERSHIP

In full KFSN tradition, with its emphasis on encouraging graduates to become innovative, groundbreaking leaders, Deloras Plake Jones, class of '63, was appointed the first Kaiser Permanente California and Health System chief nursing executive. Jones was one of many nurse leaders who paved the way to elevating the nursing profession's role and influence in health care. She, along with other graduates, has been a model of KFSN's legacy of leadership learnings that maintain their relevance today:

- Aligning proposed innovations to an organization's overarching mission and vision
- Being bold, taking calculated risks, nurturing collegial relationships and practicing self-care
- Identifying talent and empowering nurses to think critically, innovate and practice in ways that challenge the norm and promote evidence-based approaches to value-added care
- Incorporating values-based leadership at all levels of the organization, placing a high value on diversity, advanced education, professional practice and interprofessional collaboration
- Envisioning care beyond the traditional acute care settings, with a focus on innovative possibilities to promote wellness, prevent illness and support healthy communities

The more than 1,000 KFSN graduates immeasurably enhanced the nursing profession and the quality of and approach to health care delivery nationwide; KFSN nurses continue to shape nursing care now and for the future.

KAISER PERMANENTE NURSING IN 2020

It's hard to overstate the impact of the countless innovations and pioneering efforts of KFSN graduates and early KP nurses on KP's care environments today. The political, social and economic challenges of the current environment are vastly different than those of the 1940s, yet they echo nursing's enduring call to action as champions of access, affordability and high-quality care for all.

Early KP nurses might well be awed by how Kaiser Permanente looks 75 years later, having advanced well beyond its humble and often turbulent beginnings. Kaiser Permanente now provides integrated health care services to more than 12 million members across eight geographic regions, offering community-based care in 39 hospitals and 700 medical and outpatient facilities. Little could the nurse pioneers imagine that KP nurses would number 63,000, and that — working in close partnership with 22,000 physicians — KP would achieve national recognition for excellence in compassionate integrated care, transformational leadership, research, policy and quality clinical outcomes.[21]

ADVANCING KP NURSING TODAY

A 2016 graphic representation of key milestones, produced by Marilyn Chow, former vice president and chief nurse executive for KP National Patient Care Services (NPCS), offers a glimpse into the many advancements in KP nursing today.[22] The pace of continuous nursing innovation and health systems transformation has accelerated further under the visionary leadership of Linda Knodel, senior vice president for NPCS since 2017.

Knodel championed the renewal of KP's Nursing Professional Practice Model, helping reaffirm the central role Kaiser nurses have in transforming professional practice and leading interdisciplinary care delivery across the enterprise.[23] Systems leaders and clinical nurses across all eight KP regions are advancing the discipline and practice of professional nursing while continually innovating patient-family-centered care and building for nursing's future.

KP's nursing workforce makes up the largest professional sector in KP today — and KP is led by Chairman and CEO Greg Adams, who is a nurse. KP nurses are an expansive transformational force for embedding and sustaining clinical excel-

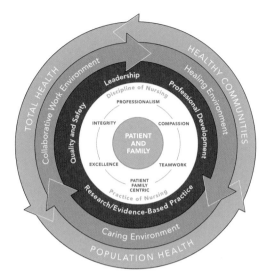

THE KAISER PERMANENTE NURSING VISION

As leaders, clinicians, researchers, innovators and scientists, Kaiser Permanente nurses are advancing the delivery of excellent, compassionate care for our members across the continuum, and boldly transforming care to improve the health of our communities and nation.

Extraordinary nursing care.
Every patient.
Every time.

KAISER PERMANENTE.

lence and operational best practices that differentiate highly reliable organizations from all others. The original vision of Dr. Garfield included a future where KP nurses, practicing within an integrated care model and equipped with the most advanced education and clinical preparation, would help ensure KP could advance and spread the influence of its total health mission effectively. KFSN graduates and KP nurses throughout KP's history have helped the organization deliver on its mission; they now are serving as the present-day knowledge workers, solution seekers and champions of quality patient care and world-class nursing services.[24] True to the KFSN ideals and despite quantum advancements in scientific knowledge, pharmacotherapy and state-of-the art technology over the years, KP nurses and teams remain grounded in KFSN ideals of high-quality patient care that integrates the most timely and sophisticated "high-tech interventions" while continually ensuring the patient remains at the center of everything, and that "high-touch care" is delivered by compassionate and highly qualified nurses and interprofessional teams.[25]

THE KP NURSE SCHOLARS ACADEMY: A TRIBUTE TO KFSN EXCELLENCE

The launch of the KP Nurse Scholars Academy (NSA) in 2015 is just one example of a bold initiative and trajectory for advancing academic preparation, evolving nursing professionalism and nurturing future nurse leaders at all levels of

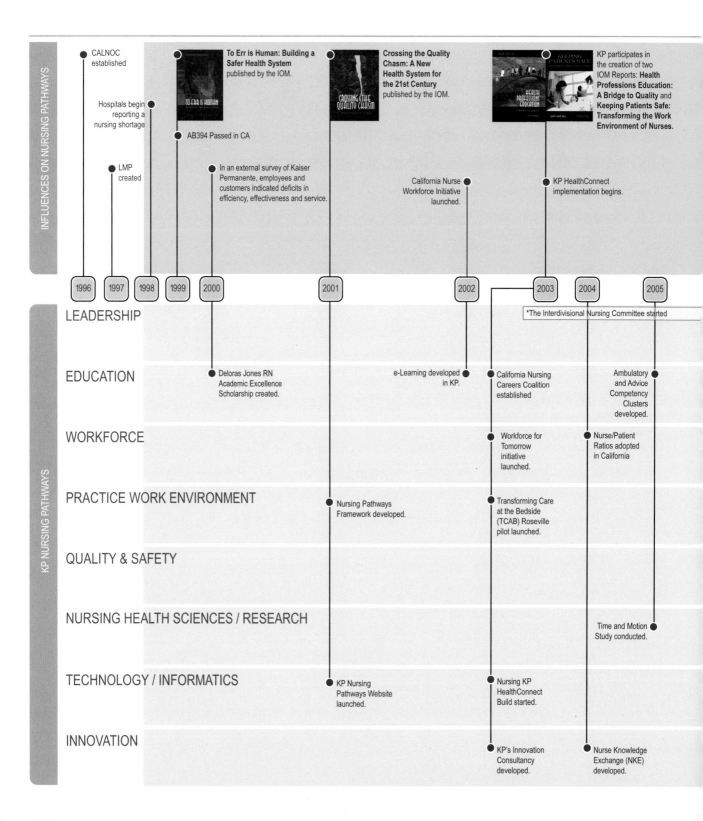

INFLUENCES ON NURSING PATHWAYS

- CALNOC established
- Hospitals begin reporting a nursing shortage
- LMP created
- AB394 Passed in CA
- **To Err is Human: Building a Safer Health System** published by the IOM.
- In an external survey of Kaiser Permanente, employees and customers indicated deficits in efficiency, effectiveness and service.
- **Crossing the Quality Chasm: A New Health System for the 21st Century** published by the IOM.
- California Nurse Workforce Initiative launched.
- KP participates in the creation of two IOM Reports: **Health Professions Education: A Bridge to Quality** and **Keeping Patients Safe: Transforming the Work Environment of Nurses.**
- KP HealthConnect implementation begins.

1996 | 1997 | 1998 | 1999 | 2000 | 2001 | 2002 | 2003 | 2004 | 2005

KP NURSING PATHWAYS

LEADERSHIP
- *The Interdivisional Nursing Committee started

EDUCATION
- Deloras Jones RN Academic Excellence Scholarship created.
- e-Learning developed in KP.
- California Nursing Careers Coalition established
- Ambulatory and Advice Competency Clusters developed.

WORKFORCE
- Workforce for Tomorrow initiative launched.
- Nurse/Patient Ratios adopted in California

PRACTICE WORK ENVIRONMENT
- Nursing Pathways Framework developed.
- Transforming Care at the Bedside (TCAB) Roseville pilot launched.

QUALITY & SAFETY

NURSING HEALTH SCIENCES / RESEARCH
- Time and Motion Study conducted.

TECHNOLOGY / INFORMATICS
- KP Nursing Pathways Website launched.
- Nursing KP HealthConnect Build started.

INNOVATION
- KP's Innovation Consultancy developed.
- Nurse Knowledge Exchange (NKE) developed.

KP Nursing Milestones: 1996 - 2016

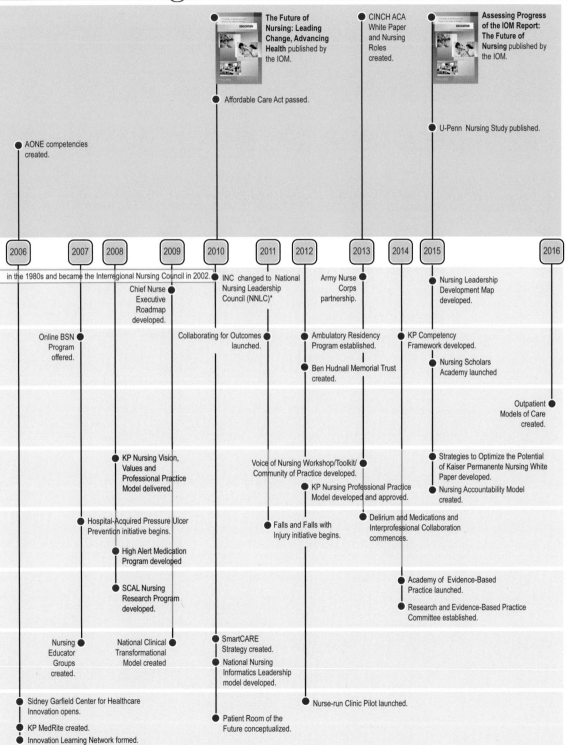

The Future of Nursing: Leading Change, Advancing Health published by the IOM.

CINCH ACA White Paper and Nursing Roles created.

Assessing Progress of the IOM Report: The Future of Nursing published by the IOM.

Affordable Care Act passed.

U-Penn Nursing Study published.

AONE competencies created.

| 2006 | 2007 | 2008 | 2009 | 2010 | 2011 | 2012 | 2013 | 2014 | 2015 | | 2016 |

in the 1980s and became the Interregional Nursing Council in 2002.

INC changed to National Nursing Leadership Council (NNLC)*

Army Nurse Corps partnership.

Nursing Leadership Development Map developed.

Chief Nurse Executive Roadmap developed.

Online BSN Program offered.

Collaborating for Outcomes launched.

Ambulatory Residency Program established.

KP Competency Framework developed.

Ben Hudnall Memorial Trust created.

Nursing Scholars Academy launched

Outpatient Models of Care created.

KP Nursing Vision, Values and Professional Practice Model delivered.

Voice of Nursing Workshop/Toolkit/Community of Practice developed.

Strategies to Optimize the Potential of Kaiser Permanente Nursing White Paper developed.

KP Nursing Professional Practice Model developed and approved.

Nursing Accountability Model created.

Hospital-Acquired Pressure Ulcer Prevention initiative begins.

High Alert Medication Program developed

Falls and Falls with Injury initiative begins.

Delirium and Medications and Interprofessional Collaboration commences.

SCAL Nursing Research Program developed.

Academy of Evidence-Based Practice launched.

Research and Evidence-Based Practice Committee established.

Nursing Educator Groups created.

National Clinical Transformational Model created

SmartCARE Strategy created.

National Nursing Informatics Leadership model developed.

Sidney Garfield Center for Healthcare Innovation opens.

Nurse-run Clinic Pilot launched.

KP MedRite created.

Patient Room of the Future conceptualized.

Innovation Learning Network formed.

the organization who can respond to the complex issues of health care in a new age of health care reform. NSA is aligned to the Institutes of Medicine (IOM) Future of Nursing workforce goals, which include achieving 80 percent baccalaureate or higher education, doubling the number of doctoral-prepared nurses, prioritizing workforce diversity, and increasing clinical and academic faculty.[26]

KP Northern California senior leadership embraced the IOM's recommendations and funded the NSA to offer RN-BSN, master's and doctoral nursing programs to elevate professional practice and prepare nurses to serve as change agents at all levels of the organization.

The academy intentionally expanded upon KFSN core values, forging new academic clinical partnerships with reputable universities that demonstrated shared values and strong commitments to diversity. Curriculum has been co-created to ensure theory-guided integration of caring science, ethics, evidence-based clinical and leadership best practices, research, social justice, community service and the essentials of self-care to foster nurses' resilience.

These unprecedented community-based partnerships were recognized nationally by the American Association of Colleges of Nursing for Exemplary Academic Practice Partnership in 2018.[27] NSA has established as a strategic priority cultivating the hearts and minds of nurses at all levels to realize the vision of transforming self and systems, and to foster a culture of disruptive innovation and creative solutions for today's health care challenges.

KP'S CULTURE OF EXCELLENCE: THE PURSUIT OF MAGNET

The pursuit of the American Nurses Credentialing Center's prestigious Magnet® Hospital Designation, first achieved by KP Irvine Medical Center in 2017[28] and then by KP Anaheim Medical Center in 2018,[29] is a focused organizational priority that reflects KP's longstanding commitment and ongoing investment as champions of nursing excellence. A University of Pennsylvania study in 2016 identified that KP's nursing and performance metrics meet and often exceed those of existing Magnet Hospitals across the nation, identifying that KP's investment in nursing, patient-centered care and organizational culture is one of its greatest differentiators in achieving highly reliable, safe, quality patient care outcomes.[30]

ENVISIONING THE FUTURE: SUSTAINING THE LEGACY

This book pays loving tribute to the spirit of KFSN graduates and early Kaiser nurses and to their dedication to professional nursing. Their collective knowledge, wisdom and voice informs and transforms KP nursing every day.

The earliest KP nurses and KFSN graduates lived out their passion for nursing while serving a noble mission and creating a vision of total health for all. This tireless and remarkable dedication to patient-family-centered care and clinical excellence resulted in an indelible contribution and sustained impact on KP nursing which thrives through the dynamic, creative, often disruptive and enduring spirit of every KP nurse past, present and well into the future.[31]

The future of nursing in KP remains bright, and the advancements we envision today ultimately will serve to strengthen and evolve our shared legacy of extraordinary care for every patient, every time, for generations to come.[32]

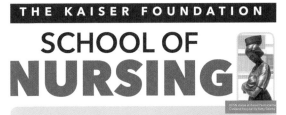

THE KAISER FOUNDATION
SCHOOL OF NURSING

At the end of World War II when the Permanente health plan opened to the public, qualified nurses were in short supply. Kaiser Permanente's founding physician Sidney Garfield, MD, articulated his hope for the future in the Second Annual Report of the Permanente Foundation Hospital in 1945:

"We have mentioned previously our conviction that teaching and training is essential to quality maintenance.... We are planning an accredited school of nursing which will be free from the traditional pressure of economics on nursing education and permit proper emphasis and time in the purely medical aspects of instruction, carrying this on to nursing specialization in the various fields and medical care on a parallel with resident physician training in medicine."

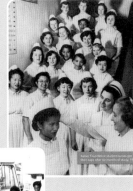

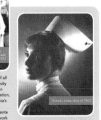

The Permanente School of Nursing became the Kaiser Foundation School of Nursing when it became independent from the hospital in 1953.

In 1947 the Permanente Foundation established a school of nursing to train more nurses and help alleviate the shortage.

Over the decades, strong leadership and high academic standards earned the school a reputation as an exemplary institution. From the beginning, students took general education and science courses at nearby College of Holy Names in Oakland and Contra Costa College in El Sobrante; this allowed them to earn credits that were transferable to a four-year college where they could pursue higher degrees.

The school was noted for its recruitment of students that represented the diversity of the community - this set it apart from most others at that time in California.

The school became independent from the hospital in 1953, changing the name from the Permanente School of Nursing to the Kaiser Foundation School of Nursing. At that time, the students were no longer used for staffing the hospital, and their clinical experiences were thus related to what they were learning in the classroom.

Student scores in State Board Examinations the 1960s and 1970s

consistently ranked in the top three of all California programs, including university schools. KFSN students participated in clinical rotation programs in rehabilitation, community, and rural health. California's first nurse practitioners were trained there by physicians from The Permanente Medical Group so they could better work in a pre-paid healthcare system that focused on prevention and wellness.

In 1976, the school graduated its last class, as the Board of Trustees was unsuccessful in developing a partnership with a four-year college to offer a baccalaureate degree in nursing. Over a period of 30 years, 1,065 nurses were educated at the school of nursing.

The legacy of KFSN continues through an active alumni association which grants scholarships to nursing students. Alumni and the Kaiser Permanente Nurse Scholars Academy produced an award-winning video, The Legacy of Nursing, Honoring Our Past, and a nurse sculpture honoring the KFSN graces the patio outside the Kaiser Permanente Oakland hospital.

KAISER PERMANENTE.

COVID-19: A New Page in Nursing's History

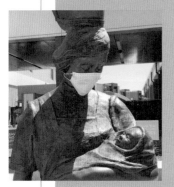

As we finalize this loving tribute to the history of the Kaiser Foundation School of Nursing, intended as a source of celebration and inspiration for all nurses during "2020: The Year of the Nurse and the Midwife," KP nurses and interdisciplinary care teams are battling a devastating pandemic now known as COVID-19.

Guided by the relevant and revered traditions of Florence Nightingale, nurses everywhere are caring for a vulnerable global community with extraordinary professionalism, dedication, courage, compassion and data-informed interventions. The heroic efforts of KP nurses exemplify the very best of nursing as highly-skilled clinicians, educators, leaders, researchers, innovators, and scientists. We remain in constant awe of their devotion to the profession and tireless efforts to provide excellent patient and family-centered care during the most challenging and strenuous of circumstances.

Through the heroic efforts of nurses across the enterprise and around the world, lives are being spared, patients and families comforted, and a grateful public is reassured that nurses persevere on the front lines while communities remain actively quarantined and steadily progress toward recovery and healing. This tragic health crisis vividly demonstrates that nurses everywhere are best prepared for these critical moments in history — as they have been across time — when the hallowed calling to serve, protect and care for those at risk or afflicted remains foremost in their hearts and minds. Nurses truly shine as beacons of trust and hope for humanity.

The landscape of healthcare and nursing in the 21st century will be deeply impacted by the events unfolding during the printing of this book and we take heart in knowing nurses will lead the essential transformation of systems, patient care and policy through new and disruptive innovations that strengthen the values of total health, prevention, access, quality, and affordability of healthcare for generations to come.

We extend our heartfelt gratitude to every nurse who paved the way, answered the call, held a hand and sacrificed their all for the welfare of those entrusted to their care. You remain a continued source of inspiration for these writings and we celebrate your indomitable spirit of love, compassion, and wisdom as we face the challenges required to co-create the future and give voice to the yet untold chapters of nursing's history and cherished contributions together.

Linda Knodel, RN

Senior Vice President/Chief Nurse Executive

Kaiser Permanente National Patient Care Services

Deloras Jones, RN

Jim D'Alfonso, RN

Editors

YEAR OF THE
NURSE
2020
LEAD · INNOVATE · EXCEL
ANA ENTERPRISE

Bernard Tyson
with maquette when
the KFSN Alumni
Association gifted
it to him for his
support of the
sculpture, c. 2017.

APPENDIX

Philosophy of Kaiser Foundation School of Nursing

The philosophy of KFSN circa 1962 (the DNA of KFSN) illustrates how the primary objectives of the school emerged.

It is our belief that:

- The practice of Nursing includes maintenance of health, individual care of the patient, and education of the patient to care for himself.

- Education is a continuous process whereby the individual learns through experience to think critically and when necessary to change behavior patterns to those which are personally and socially acceptable.

- Critical thinking is the process of defining problems, formulating objectives, searching out scientific principles, instituting a course of action and objectively evaluating the results.

- Nursing education is a process which has as it[s] basis a body of knowledge which is both art and science and which provides learning situation[s] of a continuous nature to prepare practitioners to fulfill nursing needs. These learning situations are under the direction of a Faculty Organization whose members are considered to be qualified by current standards of the profession.

- An atmosphere which allows for individual expression and participation in group activities is desirable for learning.

- It is the responsibility of the Faculty Organization to recommend physical facilities conducive to learning.

- Each member of the Faculty Organization must be willing and able to grasp new concepts and to make necessary changes in attitude and action.

- Research is an integral part of a sound educational program.

Methodology

When I was asked to speak about the history and legacy of the Kaiser Foundation School of Nursing at the 2015 dedication of the sculpture at the Oakland Medical Center, I began doing some research. History was easy to find — there is a treasure trove of material in the Kaiser Permanente Archives. But what is a legacy?

I learned a legacy is what you are remembered for after you're gone. How does it relate to the history of the school? As the Alumni Association Board of Directors, the Legacy Committee and I began digging into the archives and listened to what alumni were saying about what was so important to them about KFSN, some themes began developing.

We then thought about what was occurring in the profession at this time — how the Patient Protection and Affordable Care Act was redefining how health care needed to be delivered, how this influenced the emerging role of the nurse, and how nurse educators were struggling with preparing new nurses to practice in this evolving health care environment. The legacy of KFSN started to unfold.

The way we were trained as Kaiser students is just what was being called for in new roles for nurses today, and the way we were educated is what schools of nursing are faced with today as they prepare nurses for these roles. How did this relate to KFSN — our history and our legacy?

The more we learned about our legacy, the more we thought we had a story to tell. We needed to write a book about our school of nursing. Jim D'Alfonso, DNP, RN, PhD(h), NEA-BC, FNAP, Executive Director, Regional Patient Care Services & KP Nurse Scholars Academy, Kaiser Foundation Hospitals/Health Plan felt the story revealed the foundation of nursing within Kaiser Permanente and was related to the pillars of the recently established Nurse Scholars Academy, designed to prepare KP's nurse leaders.

Furthermore, he thought our story was one that described "disruptive innovation" in education and practice. He became our champion for the book. D'Alfonso wanted all Kaiser nurses to hear our story, to learn about their roots and heritage as Kaiser nurses. He also thought we had a story to tell to those outside of the organization — to nurse educators, to nurse leaders and to the profession as a whole.

We tested this hypothesis via a 2018 Nursing Administration Quarterly article titled "Kaiser School of Nursing: A 70-Year Legacy of Disruptive Innovation." The response to the article told us we were on the right track — others wanted to hear our story.

To get started, we needed to learn from our alumni what they thought made KFSN unique and set it apart from other schools at the time, and to capture their stories. Kaiser historian Steve Gilford enthusiastically signed on and got the process under way. He had researched the histories of Henry J. Kaiser and Kaiser Permanente and had written much about both — and he thought the story of the school of nursing was a gap in the Kaiser history that he was eager to close.

We sent a questionnaire to all known alumni to launch the writing of the book. More than 80 of them responded, providing rich information from which to build our collective story. Some of these alumni then were interviewed to provide their oral histories, with an eye toward stories that represented the decades and notable periods of the school's history. We also interviewed alumni and others who could offer a balance in the telling of the KSFN story. In all, over 40 oral histories were captured. Everyone who contributed to this book gave us their approval, allowing us to use their comments.

Remarkably, what emerged from the interviews and videos were themes from throughout the school's 30-year history — themes that became the legacy elements, those aspects of the school that made it different from others schools of nursing and whose relevance have reemerged in what is important in the practice and education of nurses today.

The repetition of these themes was the reinforcement needed to describe the legacy elements.

Grounding the history and the description of the legacy elements was a book written by Judith Dunning, which captured the oral history of Clair O'Sullivan Lisker, class of '51A. "Clair Lisker: A Voice for Nursing Education, Kaiser Permanente, 1948–1991," was rich in historical details and became an important resource in connecting the stories told by alumni and documenting the legacy elements. As Lisker had graduated in the second class, stayed on as faculty and later became associate director of the school, she touched the lives of all 1,065 graduates.

Books written by Dr. John Smilley and Tom Debley, the rich material derived from the Kaiser Permanente Archives included photos and research provided by Lincoln Cushing, Steve Gilford's personal historical interviews with Kaiser Permanente leaders, and a video produced by KP's Multimedia Department for MaryAnn Thode in 2007 about KFSN also served as invaluable resources for this manuscript.

In 2016, KP Northern California Region Multimedia Communications produced two videos that recorded the voices of KFSN Alumni that helped connect the legacy of KFSN to the pillars of the Nurse Scholars Academy: "Memorable Care Experiences" and "Honoring Out Past." The latter video received the 2017 Bronze Telly award in the nonbroadcast production history category (www.kp.org.nursescholarsacademy/story/legacy).

An editorial board representing alumni helped ensure the book was connected to the Alumni Association and provided critical feedback to the author. Terri Moss provided the editorial support and overall direction and oversight needed to bring the book to fruition and ensuring appropriate editorial, graphic and printing resources were available to accomplish our task.

— Deloras Jones,
    Class of '63, President, KFSN Alumni Association

2020 Kaiser Foundation School of Nursing Alumni Association Board of Directors

Deloras Jones, *President*

Deana Medinas, *Vice President*

Pat Rodrigues, *Secretary*

Joan Carr, *Treasurer*

Marian Feinstein, *Assistant Treasurer*

Rebecca Calloway

Clair Lisker

Phyllis Moroney

Susie Pinckard

Helen Robinson

The Legacies of the Kaiser Foundation School of Nursing

KFSN was an innovator in how nurses were educated, driven by the desire to train nurses to implement and integrate the Permanente way of practicing medicine into Kaiser Permanente's care delivery model:

- Autonomous school, separate from the training hospital, with its own board of trustees and funding source, and freedom to define the education provided.

- Curriculum drove clinicals and hands-on learning, not the need to staff the hospital; clinical education and lectures went hand in hand.

- Diversity of student body and inclusion; no discrimination in admitting students.

- Learned "zero" tolerance for discrimination in providing health care and the belief that all individuals deserve quality care regardless of their color or ethnicity.

- Advanced education and academic partners provided fully transferable college credit toward a baccalaureate degree in nursing.

- Continuation of learning was an expectation that promoted the importance of lifelong learning.

- Interprofessional education through lectures provided by The Permanente Medical Group physicians covering the medical aspects of illness or disease, and including student nurses on patient rounds along with medical residents.

- Clinical rotations went beyond the hospital to where the patients were receiving care, providing for continuity of patient care — whether in the clinic or at home, or in a rehab center or psych facility.

- Critical thinking was the foundation of how the students were taught, with research supporting what was learned (evidence-based practice).

- Taught to be leaders in whatever field the graduate went into, whether clinical practice, education or administration, or became innovators in health care delivery.

- Professional confidence and accountability enabled one to expand her/his reach into expanded roles and opportunities that made an impact on the health of communities.

- Well-prepared faculty, many with higher degrees, were given the autonomy and encouragement to try out new ways of teaching students; they modeled professional attributes for nursing students.

- Learned to create an integrated approach to the healing environment, through the art and the skill to "care" for the whole patient and family, and to provide individualized care.

- Applied holistic aspects of nursing care with a focus on the individual and family-centered care.

- Learned to be an integral member of a team, working with members of other services and disciplines, as colleagues to physicians, and contributors to the care of patients and the health of the community as part of a team effort.

- Cultural and social development with a focus on work-life balance leading to a well-rounded individual and minimizing burnout.

- Self-care, as a foundation for nursing others by caring for one's self.

- A flourishing sense of community that built long-lasting friendships and pride in the school.

- Taught to implement the Permanente way of practicing medicine (now known as Permanente Medicine) — prevention, wellness and patient education, all in a prepaid integrated health care delivery system with group practice.

- Innovation in education and health care was a hallmark that was evident throughout the history of the school, which mirrored the evolution of Kaiser Permanente.

Honoring Our Faculty

More than 80 responses from questionnaires and 41 oral history interviews carried a strong, resonating theme emphasizing the impact our instructors had on each graduate.

As we celebrate the legacy of the Kaiser Foundation School of Nursing, we celebrate our faculty — some of whom were KFSN graduates. It was our faculty who made the school what it was and shaped its legacy elements. It was the faculty who made our school the "disruptive innovator" in nursing education, which was reflected in each alumni's career choice and professional practice.

We honor our faculty for their fabulous work in creating an exceptional school of nursing, and developing a cohort of 1,065 registered nurses over 30 years whose impact on nursing continues to be felt to this day.

- You created the environment that enabled us to excel by teaching us how to become a nurse — not just academically or in clinical skills, but in teaching us how to actualize the heart and soul of nursing — the caring for our patients.

- You taught us how to think critically; how to incorporate patient education into patient care; how to treat and care for the whole patient and their families — long before holistic health was popular.

- You taught us to be confident and armed us with leadership skills that enabled all new graduates to confidently walk into their first new jobs knowing what was expected of a nurse.

- You taught us how to make beds with mitered corners, to give comforting back rubs, to act like a lady, and to use proper etiquette when smoking a cigarette.

- You taught us how to respectfully interact with physicians, but not in a subordinate manner; how to give an injection that did not hurt and how to comfort a frightened child; and how to implement the Permanente way of practicing medicine — even if you did not know you were doing that at the time.

- You coached, tutored and supported students through the decades to ensure our success. You modeled how to interact with patients and families. And you were at our side when we encountered patient interactions that left indelible impressions in our minds — usually our first dramatic patient experience.

- You ensured our clinicals were aligned with our lectures. While we were not staffing the hospital, when we worked in the hospital for pay as students, you were there when we needed you.

- Within the framework and latitude you had with the Board of Trustees and the directors of the school, you tried new and innovative ways to educate us — either in our clinicals or approaches to our curriculum.

- Our academic achievements were evident in state board exam scores where we consistently ranked in the top three schools of nursing in the state.

We were educated in an environment that laid the foundation for our continuing educational pursuits and professional lives and achievements. This was evident by what so many of our graduates did after graduating, whether we attained advanced degrees and applied our nursing in educational, practice and administrative roles, or in our exemplary roles as clinical nurses in a variety of settings. We were able to practice the career we loved, expressing the heart and soul of nursing.

KFSN Alumni

Year	First, Middle, Maiden Name	Last (known) Name
50	BETTY BAUM	PREVATT
50	BETTY FOWLER	MESHKE
50	CAROL CRONE	ADAMS
50	CLARA THOMAS	JOHNSTON
50	DORRIS FACEY	LOVRIN
50A	FRANCES WEIR	AMMERMAN
50	GENEVEVE RIVAS	GORRELL
50	GEORGETTE KURTZ	KIRBY
50	JEANNE OREY	ABBOTT
50	LORAE WORT	HUDSON
50	MARY MOORE	IVEY
50	NORMA APRILANTI	RUGG
50	RUTH BALLERT	MARTIN
50	RUTH SUNESON	NYQUIST
50	VIRGINIA CAREY	MORE
50	YVONNE SIEMERS	MARTH
51B	ANNALOU BEZPALEC	JOHANSSON
51A	BARBARA MIMMS	PARKS
51B	BARBARA WAGNER	KYHN
51B	CANDIDA BARCELLOS	MC KENZIE
51	CARNATION MANILAG	BANSUELO
51A	CAROL GIFFORD	MC MURRAY
51B	CATHLEEN TAYLOR	GRIFFIN
51	CHARLOTTE STARK	SPECK
51A	CLAIR O'SULLIVAN	LISKER
51B	CRUZITA CRUZ	YBARRA
51A	DIANE LaFOND	MARLER
51A	DOROTHY JEAN KREGER	MC LAUGHLIN
51 B	ELLEN BODENHAMER	DARCY
51B	ELSIE HUNTINGTON	MAYES
51B	ESTHER DOTTS	LARSON
51	GRACE KELLAR	WILSON
51B	HAZEL GUILINGER	COX
51B	JEAN HAAG	HARPER
51A	JOSEPHINE	BUECHLEY
51A	JOYCE BUGBEE	COPPINI
51	LILLIAN BUTLER	BURNHAM
51B	LORRAINE LYCKLAMA	CHILDERS
51A	MARGARET ADDISON	PRICE
51A	MARIAN SMITH	TRAUB
51A	MARION DOOLAN	FYFE
51A	MARY JANE ON	CHAN
51A	MAYROSE V.	MELL
51A	NADINE SNOW	SPURRIER
51A	NANCY HORIE	SUDA
51B	PATRICIA ANN	RYAN
51	PATRICIA BERGSTROM	EAKLE
51A	PATRICIA WARD	RALSTON
51	PAULINE KOSOBUSKI	ROUSE
51B	ROBERTA SMITH	NEARY
51	SARA LEMAN	BINGHAM
51	SUZUIA KIRITANI	SHOLES
51A	VALERIE BABB	MASIEL
51B	VALERIE LEWIS	SAMELSON
51B	VERDIA LOU WILLIAMS	PERRY
51A	VIRGINIA LAWRENCE	FORSETH
51	VIVIENNE LAVERNE	CORTNER
52A	ALLANA SMITH	CORBAT
52B	BARBARA BASISTA	WOODY
52	BARBARA JUNE	SPARKMAN
52	BARBARA ZIMMERMAN	CLARK
52B	BETTY JO CATO	BOTZBACH
52B	CAROLYN ROOD	WESSELS
52	ELIZABETH OREY	TRAVERS
52	FUMIE FUJIMOTO	LEE
52	JANETTE LORRAINE	STECKBAR
52	KATHLEEN FISHER	COULTER
52B	KATHRYN DUGAN	MOZZETTI
52B	LESLIE RAGGIO	KAPPLER
52	MARJORIE BUNGE	MILLER
52	MARJORIE CUNDALL	BABB
52B	MARLENE TOKES	JONES
52A	MARY CAMERON	RICA
52	MARY MASON	BUNGE
52	MIRIAM KAPLAN	KIRSCHNER
52	MONTE DEWEY	BARNHART
52	NANCY HELENE	ALLEN
52	NANCY RUTH	PHILLIPS
52	ZELLA ST MARTIN	TAYLOR
53	ALICIA REYNA	MC ATEE
53B	ARLENE BASISTA	VAN NORDEN
53	BEEBE PAOE	MOORE
53	BERTHA FOO	NG
53	BOBBIE	ANGELL
53B	CAROLYN CHIRSTEN	SPIKER
53	CLAIR KING	MC CAMEY
53	DELORIS ROBERTS	FREDSON
53B	DOROTHY SHEINBERG	RENSTROM
53B	ETHEL O'DONNELL	MORGAN
53	GERRAINE HULEN	HOYT
53	INGE	DE LA CAMP
53B	IRENE MILLER	GOODISON
53	JAN REILLY	BASALTO
53	JANET RABE	MITCHELL
53B	JERALYN WADE	FISHER
53B	JOANN RASMUSSEN	KIEFER
53	JOYCE CASSADY	BIRCH
53	LOIS WALLACE	LLOYD
53B	LORIS QUINNEY	RYAN
53B	LORRAINE VARMUN	POUKISH
53B	LOWELLA MARAFFIO	ARRINGTON
53B	MADELYN ROGERS	KETCHUM
53	MARIE GEMMELL	CONTRERAS
53B	MARILYN ANDERSON	FISHER
53	MARY FISHER	SHIPLEY
53B	MARY FOSTER	BRYANT
53	MARY HUNTER	MERCER
53	MARY MARTINEZ	ALARCON
53	MASAKO SETOGUCH	NII
53	NANCY LINGARD	RICHARDSON
53	NANCY PATTERSON	HANSON
53	PATRICIA HALE	FOSTER
53	PEARL V.	KOCHERSPERGER
53	PHYLLIS WHITE	DEINES
53	SHIRLEY DIXON	BELL
53A	SHIRLEY MC FALL	GREENBANK
53	SUZANNE HILLMAN	HANSEN
53	VIRGINIA RANDOLPH	BRADSHAW
54	AMIE SHIBA	KIRITANI
54	BARBARA JANE	SCHILL
54	BERNADETTE SORA	PAULSEN
54	BETH BENSON	MILNE
54B	BETTY AVILA	FLEMER
54	BETTY STOLZMAN	SOKKAPPA
54	CAROL MARKS	DIDUR
54	CAROL PEARCY	SHOUR
54	CLARA GARNER	HARRELSON
54	CONSTANCE JAMES	ROSE
54	DIANE BOYD	CURRAN
54	DIANE EBERT	PFEFFER
54B	DOLORES MALLAN	PRYOR
54A	ELEANOR LEE	WU
54	ELIZABETH LONGSTRET	MILLER
54	ELNORA WHITE	FRANKINA
54	ESTHER BALTAZAR	BUTTIGIG
54	GEORGIA MAE	SMITH
54	GERALDINE ANNE	WELLS
54	GERTRUDE MACNAB	VAN ATTA
54	HELEN SCHEUERMANN	HARWARD
54	JANET WILLETT	HAGGART
54B	JANICE BARTELS	NEWBURN

54	JANIS HORTON	MOCETTINI	
54	JERRY BARMORE	HOGAN	
54	JESSIE HEAD	CUNNINGHAM	
54B	JOANNE HUTSON	KAMINSKI	
54B	JOYCE MILLER	NIKKEL	
54	JUANITA PRESWOOD	KING	
54	LA VERNE DOLORES	OYARZO	
54	LAURA GALL	RODELANDER	
54	LETTIE THOMAS	ERICSON	
54	MABEL OUSHANA	FRANKLIN	
54	MARGUERITE NICKERSO	CHAPMAN	
54	MARIA ARCHIBEOUE	SMITH	
54	MARIANNE CROW	POMEROY	
54B	MARILYNN PADDOCK	BRANDMEYER	
54	MARLENE STONE	MITCHELL	
54	MARTHA LAYCOCK	LOPER	
54	MARY DEICHELBOHRER	HANNON	
54	MARY KATHRYN	EVANS	
54	MARV MCCONNELL	EASLEY	
54	MORRIE PAYNE	MATTHEW	
54A	NAOMI EIKO	TANIKAWA	
54A	RITA BOPP	CARROLL	
54A	RITA HUCKO	DIETZ	
54	ROSE SNOW	SKAGGS	
54	ROSIE	GUTIERREZ	
54B	ROWENE MC KENZIE	BISHOP	
54	RUTH FORESTER	MARYATT	
54A	RUTH FREEMAN	FRANKLIN	
54	VERNETTE DALE	STARK	
54B	WILMA BEAVERS	BUJACK	
54A	YUKIE HURIE	GOISHI	
55	ALICE GUTIEREZ	MULVANEY	
55B	ALICE RAYMOND	FLURY	
55	ALMA HIROSE	MILLER	
55A	ANNABELLE FRAZIER	WHIPPLE	
55	ANNE WEAVER	HOGENSON	
55B	AVICE HATTON	TAYLOR	
55A	BARBARA PERRIN	ZAKI	
55A	BETTIE HENDERSON	EATCHEL	
55B	BETTY SAXBY	KRAEMER	
55B	BEVERLY PEART	FURNISH	
55A	CLARISE POLLARD	BERGQUIST	
55B	DONNA LURVEY	FRASIER	
55	DONNA MAE	HILSCHER	
55A	DORIS HONEYCUTT	FOLK	
55B	DOROTHY MAINES	CAREY	
55A	DOROTHY THOMAS	HACKETT	
55	EDITH GAMBLE	CROFORT	
55B	EMILY M.	THOMANN	

55B	EVA CONLEY	FLOHR	
55B	FRANCES MAIER	HEDRICK	
55	GLORIA PITTS	MANOR	
55B	IRIS GROVE LAWRENCE	MANFRE	
55B	JANICE WILSON	SATER	
55	JOSEPHINE MOVO	OSBORNE	
55A	LA VERNE POWELL	SNIDER	
55B	LORRAINE MARKLEY	TUDOR	
55B	MARGARET HAMACNI	SHIMADA	
55B	MARGARET TARP-	WATCHERS	
55A	MARILYN NYSTROM	AIKEN	
55	MARY SULLIVAN	DALY	
55B	MARYLOU BRENNAN	GORMLY	
55B	MILDA LARCHE	GREENBAUM	
55B	MILDRED GORRE	EWING	
55B	PATRICIA FOY	NIEMEYER	
55	PATRICIA SIMMONS	HOLLAND	
55B	PATRICIA STEWART	SCHUSTER	
55B	PRENETTA HARRIS	TODD	
55	PRISALLA PURSE	BARNS	
55	RICA KOST	ANDERSON	
55B	ROBERTA IRISH	WILSON	
55A	SETSUKO MIYADA	TAKEMORI	
55B	SYLVIA HOGUE	IVY	
55B	VIRGINIA	GROTH	
56	BARBARA HALL	EDMAN	
56	BARBARA KEATOR	MAUSER	
56	CARLETHA JANE	NEWKIRK	
56	CAROLE PEARCE	AMOY	
56	CHARLENE BRYANT	PAPPAS	
56	CONSTANCE DA VICO	COLE	
56	CORLYN KOLSTAD	HUNTZIKER	
56	DOROTHY STREHLE	ABEE	
56	EARLYN MORGAN	LUZMOOR	
56B	EVANGELINE	FLURY	
56	HELEN KENNON	MOORE	
56	ISABELLE EMERSON	JONES	
56	JANE SAKATA	TAKEUCHI	
56	JEANNA MARY	PETERS	
56	JOANNE DUENOW	BIELEFELD	
56B	WANDA JOY LADUSAU	HAAS	
56	JOYCE GREEN	ONSTAD	
56	LOUCILE BEACHAM	MULDROW	
56A	MARCIA VAN DE MARK	GHORMLEY	
56	MARGARET CACHORA	BREEDLOVE	
56B	MARJORIE ALBAUGH	MAHNKE	
56	MARY ANN JOHNSON	EDICK	
56	MYRNA MERRILL	CLARK	
56	PATRICIA KING	FARLEY	

56	PAULA PUTNAM	JACUZZI	
56	PHYLLIS BUSSINGER	EDGAR	
56	RENEE HARDMAN	PACKARD	
56	RHEA RENNER	HOLLIDAY	
56	SARAH YORK	RIJNHOLT	
57	BARBARA BURT	SAUL	
57	BARBARA GRIFFIN	PATCHIN	
57	BETTY HAZZARD	PREVOST	
57	CAROL HENDERSON	TAMO	
57A	CAROL LYONS	TRIBBLE	
57B	CAROL SHIFTON	TAYLOR	
57B	CAROL SIEGERT	KING	
57B	CHERRILL VANDER PLOEG	CORLISS	
67	CLARITA AQUINO	ARCELLANA	
57B	DIAN KAY	WILLBUR	
57	DONNA GREEN	STANLEY	
57	DONNA MIDDAUGH	MYERS	
57	DOROTHY HOUSE	WELLS	
57	ELIZABETH FRY	PENCE	
57	EVONNE STAUSBAUGH	MC KINNEY	
57	FAYE CLEMENTS	CURRIE	
57A	FRANCES PARRA	POSADA	
57A	GERALDINE CATHERINE	CURRAN	
57B	GLENDA RIGGS	DICKINSON	
57	HELEN TANIGAWA	BEERY	
57B	JEAN BERG	MEDDAUGH	
57	JOAN GARNER	OWENS	
57	JOYCE SMITH	LARSEN	
57B	LYLLIAN LOEWEN	RUESSEGGER	
57B	LYNN DEFOREST	ROBIE	
57B	MARJORIE MEANS	MEIKLE	
57A	MARY LOUISE STEINKE	VIVIER	
57	MARY STREHLE	WIMBERLY	
57	MATTE GUILLORY	SANDER	
57	MYRA IBERA	TETERS	
57A	NANCY MORRIS	LONGHURST	
57A	NATIVIDAD JUVLAND	MUNOZ	
57	NINA CHINN	FREEMAN	
57	OFEIRA TULIAU	LUTU	
57B	PETRA LEWIS	WYNBRANDT	
57A	PHYLLIS PLANT	MORONEY	
57B	RAMONA SILVA	HODGES	
57	REPEKA ISARA	HOWLAND	
57B	SANDRA BROWN	ANDERSON	
57B	SHIRLEY JOHNSTON	KOHLMOOS	
57B	VIRGINIA	PEREZ	
57	WALLENE EISELE	CASTRO	
57	WANDA GRUBBS	HARRIS	

Year	First Name	Last Name
58	ADA LOUISE	TARKINGTON
58	AIKO	HASHIYAMA
58	ANNE DALY	HASHIYAMA
58	AUDREY LOUISE	WILLIAMS
58	BEATRICE LUCAS	COLBURN
58	BETTIE MILLER	WILLIAMS
58	BILLIE PAULINE	BRASSART
58	CAROL RICHARDSON	SHORE
58	CHRISTINA BUSEY	IRVIN
58	CONSTANCE GOTHARD	JOHNSON
58	CONSTANCE RODSETH	PORTER
58	DONNA CARPENTER	MANESS
58	GAYLE ARDEN	GORDON
58	GLADYS KASHIWAMURA	JACKSON
58	GRACE OSHITA	MIYAMOTO
58	HELEN POWELL	LOCKIE
58	JANICE SHERMAN	BERNSTEIN
58	JEAN FISHER	HARRELL
58	JEANETTE BENEDETTI	SHAW
58	JERALYN MC ELLICOTT	CARLSON
58	JOANNE BRADOVICH	WINKLE
58	JULIA BAKER	PASCUAL
58	JULIETTE WHITFIELD	POWELL
58	KATHLEEN SALT	KUKA
58	LA VONNE ROBERTS	SANFORD
58	LEONA FERRO	CAYLER
58	MARILYN RAINS	OLSWESKI
58	MAUREEN HAAG	CHESNEY
58	MARY GILLESPIE	DONE
58	MARY NAKANO	TSUKAMOTO
58	MARY ROBINSON	DURRANT
58	PEGGY HUNT	CROSS
58	SALLY	BURNHAM
58	SHARON MARIE	STOWE
58	SHIRLEY BEALS	ARMSTEAD
59	ALICE ISHIHARA	TAKAHASHI
59	BETTE YOUNGSTROM	THOMSEN
59	BETTY PAOLI	KAY
59	BEVERLY KNUTZ	COFFMAN
59	BEVERLY TOM	DECEASED 3/11/13
59	CLAUDIA COUNTS	CADWELL
59	DONNA BABBITT	KORTH
59	EDITH CRAIN	TOLBERT
59	ELEANOR GRISWOLD	GEORGE
59	EVELYN MASUMOTO	ASATO
59	FRANCES KLLLOUGH	OSBURN
59	GAIL DENNER	JONAS
59	GAYLE MAC NEIL	TAYLOR
59	GRETCHEN MUELLER	SEIFERT
59	HARRIETT PIERCE	GOODYKOONTZ
59	ILSE GAREIS	DUNCAN
59	JAN TOWNE	CONNER
59	JANICE STERN	KJELSTROM
59	JOANN WENDLAND	LESICO
59	JOSEPHINE TODD	CROSBY
59	JUANITA GALBRAITH	MITCHELL
59	LOUISE RODRIQUEZ	SPITTLE
59	LOUISE SMITH	DORIA
59	MARCIA SMITH	HUFF
59	MARLENE FLAHERTY	ROTEN
59	MARVEL CHAPMAN	NUSS
59	MARY CULLOTY	ANNONI
59	MARY KUKA	CHEEK
59	MARY LOZIER	TOLIVER
59	NATHEL PERRY	BAULDING
59	NELL THOMPSON	RANK
59	ORA SMITH	DORIA
59	ROBERTA TODD	STARSIAK
59	ROCHELLE ANDERSON	KIRKEGARRD
59	ROSALIE BELL	KING
59	ROSALIE MYERS	HEPPNER
59	ROSE FOIANINI	BIASOTTI
59	SHARON JENSEN	CUNNINGHAM
60	ANDREA BECKER	NORDSTROM
60	ARLENE TAMAKA	WAKASA
60	BARBARA DUVALL	EVERARD
60	BETTY THOMAS	JOST
60	BEVERLY JOHNS	POWELL
60	BEVERLY POWELL	KREY
60	CAROL MURRAY	STEIN
60	CAROL PINTO	VIOLET
60	CAROLE LARSON	HOCKENBARGER
60	CAROLYN TATMAN	YOUNG
60	CHRISTINA LONGANICER	MC CUNE
60	COLEEN CALHOUN	WELLS
60	(ELIZABETH) ANN MILLER	MOORE
60	ELIZABETH LOWE	HUEN
60	ELLEN WERNEGREEN	CECIL
60	EMILY ENGLISH	HARE
60	EVANGELINE JETT	CLARK
60	IDA DAVIS MC BRIDGE	PEARSON
60	IONE GRUNDSERG	LOPEZ
60	JANICE BOOTH	HOLBROOK
60	JOAN SANBORN	FROMMHAGEN
60	JOAN AASETH	BOGUE MORTIZ
60	LEONORA COFER	RUSSELL
60	LINDA FINCHAM PILE	WAITE
60	LINDA RITCHEY	SMITH
60	MARGARET ROSS	LLOYD
60	MARIE MARTHA	JOSEPH
60	MARY MILLER	WALLACE
60	MILLICENT LAMB	RIPA
60	NANCY DIRKS	SMITH
60	OLGA ELDORA	KAHLER
60	PATRICIA DOOLY	FORST
60	PATRICIA DREW	RIGNEY
60	PEARL MYERS	RICKARD
60	PEGGY PREWETT	FLEMING
60	PENELOPE SANDBERG	BELL
60	SHEILA STAFF	REILLY
60	SHERON SMITH	WARD
60	SUSAN FEARN	BRENDLEN
61	ARLENE LEBER	JECH
61	BARBARA ANDERSON	KOLBERG
61	BARBARA HARVEY	DEL ROSSO
61	BEATRICE TAYLOR	JETT
61	BENITA BRINTON	CLARK
61	BEVERLY BACHICH	WILSON
61	BEVERLY POLANICH	MOORE
61	CAROLE MAC DONALD	HEAPY
61	CLAIRE NICHOL	MARTIN
61	CONSTANCE STOHLER	HAKE
61	DEANNA	WINTER
61	ELENE GREENFELDT	BUGG
61	ESTHER SMITH	HOLMES
61	EUNICE JOAN LYNCH	KOFFLER
61	GAIL OATES	SPENCE
61	GLORIA GIBSON	MARTIN
61	GRACE DAY	ABERLE
61	IDA KRAMER	MUELLER
61	JANICE MANDEVILLE	ATKIN
61	JO ANN ADKINS	ROBINSON
61	JOYCE HITCHCOCK	GURULE
61	JUDITH GRANT	WERNER
61	KAAREN ADAMS	HAVLAN
61	LINDA YOUNG	CHAPMAN-ARTZ
61	LOIS LAWTON	ERIKSEN
61	LYNDA HAGLE	WHEELER
61	LYNNE	CROWELL
61	MARCIA MILLS	KIEFER
61	MELANIE CRAWFORD	FUNDAK
61	MYRNA ROBERTS	BOWMAN
61	PATRICIA BREUNING	BROWN
61	PATRICIA BROWNING	HOFFMAN
61	PEGGY CHURCH	MILO
61	REBECCA SCHOENTHAL	CALLOWAY
61	SALLY JO MC MARTIN	ROSENBUSCH-CLARKE

Year	Name	Surname
61	SHARON GRUBER	WALKER
61	SANDRA WOOLLEY	BERKSON
61	SHARON OTTIS	VONNEGUT
61	SHIRLEY IRWIN	STARLING
61	SUE HAMMERSMITH	MACDUFF
61	VELMA YOUNG	HAYCOCK
62	BARBARA HAOYE	FUJIMOTO
62	BARBARA WHALIN	MAKANT
62	BENITA BYRAM	DEVINE
62	BEVERLY FLURY	OSWALD
62	BILLIE THROWER	BOLDEN
62	BONNIE CALDWELL	APPLEGATE
62	BONNIE FARMER	SCUTUICK
62	CALLIE EARLENE	HENSLEE
62	CAROL LEIDECKER	MILLER
62	CAROL WILSON	GAGLIONE
62	CAROLYN ANTHONY	FISHER
62	DARRELL WOOLARD	BISKNER
62	DOROTHY FARRAR	HARMON
62	EILEEN BEAM	INGRAHAM
62	JANICE DOYEL	BENNETT
62	JOHANN ALLEN	KEYSER
62	JUDITH VAUGHAN	SMITH
62	KATHLEEN STERN	MC CARTER
62	KAY COX	WATLEY
62	LETICIA MARIANO	SACHSEL
62	LILIAN BOLDT	PRICE
62	LYRIA DE QUIS	KOLAS
62	MARILYN MC COOL	SPANGLER
62	MERETTA GREEN	SKELTON
62	PATRICIA MATSON	ABERNATHY
62	PAULA JOHNSON	YOKOYAMA
62	PAULINE RYAN	DANIEL
62	ROBERTA HAAS	QUINN
62	SANDA BERG	HUGHES
62	SANDRA HASHAGEN	TYLER
62	SANDRA SWAIN	SHEPHERD
62	SHARON LALLY	BATEN
62	SHIRLEY HEADLEY	TOMPKINS
62	SUSAN TERWILLIGER	MIRAMONTES
62	SUZANNE SPERRY	HENNINGSON
62	VERNA JEANNCH WAGGENER	SORENSON
62	WILMA NEIHEISEL	SWAN
63	BARBARA DOWD	LEONARD
63	BARBARA KRAUSE	SUPPO
63	BOBBIE FONGER	JOHNSON
63	CAROLYN CURB	HAND
63	CAROLYN KAVKA	HILLBERRY
63	CAROLYN SOUTHWORTH	NEMECEK
63	CAROL	MIDDLETON
63	COLEEN WESTCOTT	ALLEN-GOODWIN
63	CONSTANCE FIGG	CRONE
63	DELORAS PLAKE	JONES
63	DONNA WEBB	STEELE
63	DOROTHY MILLER	BROWN
63	GAY MINAMOTO	KAPLAN
63	GLENDA RIGGS	TODD
63	GLORIA VALLESCORSA	REED
63	INEZ RANDLE	MORGAN
63	JACKIE HYLTON	ANDERSON
63	JANE HOWARD	BOYCE
63	JANET FLORI	MC KIMMY
63	JANET MUELLER	CORP
63	JANICE PRICE	KLEIN
63	JOANN MODDISON	VON THUN
63	JUDITH WILSON	FIEBELKORN
63	JUDITH WITT	ROBERTS
63	KARIN MAC NEIL	LYDERS
63	KATHERINE BARLOW	TASSANO
63	LA VERA LANCE	GARDNER
63	LESLEY	MERIWETHER
63	LILA BALANON	LAKE
63	LINDA SMITH	RODRIGUES
63	LINDA WILLIAMS	PHILLIPS
63	MANUELA GIRON-CERNA	SILMAN
63	MARIAN TRETER	FEINSTEIN
63	MARIANNE GARBER	WARWICK
63	MARTHA (Norma) LEWIS	DAVIS
63	MARY JO TYLER	MARIN
63	PATRICIA BAKER	REITER
63	ROBERTA ANN	CASTRO-GREEN
63	ROBIN YUGE	TILLMAN
63	ROSEMARY LOZANO	OWENS
63	SHARON HITCHENS	ARNOLD
63	SHARON LAY	MASTERTON
63	SUSAN JONES	CARAVACA
63	WINIFRED DAVIS	BERGER
64	ANITA ANN WAGNER	GARMAN
64	ANN MARIE	SPALDING
64	ARDEN SHOPSHIRE	BRYANT
64	BEVERLY HUTT	CHOW
64	BONITA PORTER	MCFADDEN
64	CAROL ANN CAMPBELL	GRAY
64	CORNELIA SLIKKER	YOUNG
64	DARLENE PENELLI-PARKER	BUTNER
64	DONNA GODCHAUX	PORTER
64	EDDYLOU EVANS	WALLACE
64	FRANCES SORENSEN	MILLER
64	JANET HYZER	EATON
64	JANET MEYRING	JOHNSON
64	JEANNE KOLBERG	FORSTALL
64	JOAN MC NEELY	FARRAR
64	LAURIE HENRY	TITTLE
64	LEONORE	MAC ILRAITH
64	LEONA JUDSON	MONTGOMERY
64	LINDA KAY	TAYLOR
64	LOIS GROSHART	HARGRAVES
64	LORRAINE NISSEN	LEWIS
64	MARGARET CASPER	MCCULLEY
64	MARILYNN O'CONNER	BUGLER
64	MARJORIE	EDWARDS
64	MARY FLECKLIN	TURRI
64	OLGA TARASOFF	SOKOLOFF
64	PATRICIA CAROLE	GRAY
64	PATRICIA GREENE	SCHNEIDER
64	PATRICIA JOHNSON	O'CONNELL
64	PATRICIA NEWMAN	DONAHUE
64	PATRICIA SCHMIDT	REHER
64	SANDRA MC GREGOR	JANSEN
64	SANDRA STERLE	MC WILLIAMS
64	SHARON ANN	LUSHER
64	SUSAN BUTTEDAHL	DICKSON
64	SUSAN MARTIN	TUCKER
64	SUZANNE BLOMMEN	TURPIN
64	SYLVIA BARNES	BERTRAM
64	VIRGINIA MARY	NOLAN
64	VIRGINIA CRUM	ROSS
65	ALICE TICKNER	TOLLETH
65	ARLENE JAGODA	SAWYER
65	CAROL WEBSTER	SANTOR
65	CHRISTINE STEVENS	KRADJIAN
65	CLARITA WALL	WOOLDRIDGE
65	DIANA BOSON	GREER
65	DIANE ADAMS	KING
65	DONNA CLEAVES	HUNT
65	EMILY NAKAMURA	AOYAMA
65	GAIL CHRISTIAN	FORAKER
65	GAY JORDAN	CLAUSEN
65	GINGER COLTON	BJORNSTAD
65	GINNY	NOLAN
65	HELEN HARRISON	ROBINSON
65	INGRID JOHNSON	ANGST
65	JANET BRIGHT	WEAVER
65	JANICE BROWNING	POORE
65	JANNA SMITH	JENKINS
65	JEAN ANDERSON	ENOS

Year	Name	Surname
65	JEAN EPPARD	RENNER
65	KAREN DAVIES	EILERTSEN
65	KARIN SCHOENFELD	JONES
65	KATHLEEN GARRITY	CARLL
65	MARGARET CAQUATE	MONTICELLO
65	MARGARET RUDESILL	MURDOCK
65	MARY SCARCELLA	SMETEK
65	MILDRED RANGER	SCHOFIELD
65	NANCY ANN WHITE	GRUNDEL
65	NORANELL SNOWDEN	MCGILL
65	PARALUMAN MEDINA	OKIMOTO
65	PATRICIA LEISTER	WILLSON
65	PATRICIA CONRAD	KIRBY
65	PAULA MAINS	MADEHEIM
65	PENNY GRAF	SLAUGHTER
65	PRUDENCE RENAS	JENSEN
65	ROBERTA REIDY	GUIFFRE
65	SANDRA JENNINGS	HEDGPETH
65	SHARON KENT	HARRIS
65	SHARON NORDSTROM	GRINNELL
65	RALEIGH RAUDSTEIN	NOWERS
65	SUSAN SPINOLA	GEATZ
65	TAEKO AKIYOSHI	LEE
65	TONI CAMPANELLA	MACALUSO
65	VICKI ANN	BUSCH
65	VICKI MC COSKER	WHITE-SAPUTO
65	VONDA WALDREN	DERR
65	WANDA KIZZIA	PEZZAGLIA
66	ADA HAMER	GALLI
66	ANITA DRWINGA	PHILLIPS
66	ANNETTE MARIE	NELSON
66	BARBARA SORENSEN	BECK
66	CAROLYNNE EGI	MURPHY
65	CLAUDIA HERMANSON	BARSAMIAN
66	CORA ROBBINS	SCHOLL
66	DEANA CARTER	MEDINAS
66	DIANE DOSS	ARCHIBALD
66	DIANE SMITH	MATTHEW
66	ELAINE PUERTA	LAUCK
66	ELIZABETH BROWN	SCHULZE
66	FAITH THOMPSON	CASEY
66	GLORIA CAUGHEY	SCHROEDER
66	JANICE SCHNEIDER	BRADEN
66	JEAN NAKAMOTO	LAGOMARSINO
66	JEANETTE ARAKELIAN	ALTON
66	KAREN CHAPMAN	PICKARDT
66	KAREN LAEBER	RICHARDSON
66	KENDAL DEBORAH	SHARPLESS
66	LAURIE WIESINGER	PACKWOOD
66	LESA HIGH	MC BENGE
66	LILLIAN BENTLY	KARLSTRAND
66	LINDA	DIERKS
66	MARCA BARBER	DEWITT
66	MARIAN LAW	CHEUNG
66	MARY ARVEDI	BERA
66	MARY HEALY	THODE
66	MICHELE ALICATA	KITTS
66	PAMULA WARNEY	REGAN
66	PARTICIA MATSON	ABERNATHY
66	PRUDENCE BETH	SEEGER
66	SHARON WRIGHT	SANCHEZ
66	SUSAN BARTLEY	MATTSON
66	SUSAN GORANSON	RAHMEYER
66	TERUKO KONO	BURCHFIELD
66	VERNA SCHULZ	WALKER
67	BETSY WALSH	WRIGHT
67	CAROL EMRICH	PIERSON
67	CHERLE GAY	DeLONG
67	CLAIRE LOUIE	REDSTONE
67	CLAUDIA BROWN	INSKEEP
67	DIANE DOYLE	ALLEN
67	DIANE LUMSDEN	WILFERDINGER
67	DONNA MAE	ENGELS
67	EDLA KANGAS	PAPPAS
67	GERALDINE LUCAS	SALAMATIAN
67	GERALDINE VOIGHT	PIERCE
67	JANICE LEE	RENALDI
67	JO ELLEN SMITH	NYMAN
67	JOANNE JOHNSON	STONE
67	KAREN HEINEMANN	BLACK
67	KATHLEEN BENEDETTI	WESTON
67	KATHLEEN MURPHY	STEINER
67	LAUREN MCCULLOUGH	SCHEALL
67	LINDA CLARK	KERSEY
67	LINDA HANAVAN	THOMAS
67	LINDA LEE	MUSSER
67	LINDA MANSKE	NYMAN
67	MARY MODRZEJEWSKI	ROLLINS
67	MARY ANN ROSKOS	ARTHUR
67	NANCY ELLSTROM	HUVELLE
67	PEGGY ANDERSON	MEYER
67	SALLY MC DOWELL	WARNER
67	SANDRA BOYD	ATENCIO
67	SANDRA LITTRELL	NICKEL
67	SHEILA SPECK	BENSON
67	SUSAN BRALEY	ZIMMERMAN
68	BARBARA SIMS	WHITNEY
68	BONNIE DAVIS	GRUNSETH
68	CAROL KIMBROUGH	SOUSA
68	CATHERINE LESLIE	SCHUTT
68	KEATSIE S. JENSON	SWENSON
68	CLAIRE KITCHENS	MILLS
68	CLAUDIA LYNN	MOLLART
68	ELENA VICTORIA	ALBERTS
68	JACKIE DOWNS	MARTIN
68	JANET	NILSEN
68	JEAN ANNE	HOBART
68	JUANITA JEAN	FOWLER
68	JUDITH WIGLESWORTH	CHEEK
68	JULIE SIEDEL	RYDELL
68	KAREN ALLEN	ADLER
68	KATHY CLINE	HARRIS
68	CHARLENE KEATSIE	JENSEN
68	LAURETTE COLDREN	WOOD
68	LINDA IRVIN CORDOBA	GROVES
68	LINDA STRINGHAM	AVERBUCH
68	MARCIA CARROLL	STEWART
68	MARTE GILLINGHAM	THOMAS
68	MARY THOMASSEN	KECK
68	MICHELLE KINKELLA	FARRELL
68	NANCY RUTH	JOHNS
68	NANCY KELLOGG	SUMMY
68	NANCY SUTHERLAND	PETERSON
68	PATRICIA DeDOBBELEER	CRAIG
68	PATRICIA MORRISSEY	CUSTER
68	RANETTE PIKE	GIORDANO-CLARK
68	RONEALE HOSMER	DUNCAN
68	ROSE ASPEN	JACK
68	SHARON KENNEDY	ORAV
68	SUSAN GAIL	HARRIS
68	TERRY ANN	BRAWNER
68	VICTOIRE VOLF	TURNER
68	VICTORIA SOARES	FACCIUTO
69	BETSEY GERBLE	MANEE
69	CAROL	STEWART
69	CAROLE DETTLING	MING
69	CHARLOTTE MICKELBERRY	VOLF
69	CHRISRINA	COOPER
69	CHRISTINA SHOUP	MC KINSTRY
69	CINDY LOU TOMLINSON	LAGLE
69	DIANE BONOMINI	COTTI
69	DIANE EDNA	JACOBSON
69	DONNA GILLIAM	OAKLEY
69	ELAINE DRAKE	CHAR
69	ELAINE KLING	BURMAN
69	ELIZABETH DIGGS	SAINT GEORGE

Year	First Name	Surname
69	JANET LEVY	TYAS
69	JANET STEVENSON	DOUDIET
69	JOHNNIE LITSEY	THOMPSON
69	JUDITH MYERS	SEAGRAVES
69	JUDITH SMITH	SCHMIDT
69	JUDY CONWAY	AMINIAN
69	KAREN LA MANTIA	ASHIKEH
69	KATHLEEN MALONE	GARDNER
69	KRISTINE ANDERSON	ROTH
69	LINDA BIALKIN	LASHER
69	LYNDA BUBNAR	FITZHUGH
69	MARIJKE VERMEULEN	BROOKS
69	MARSHA DIANE	FOWLER
69	MARY ALICE TIRADOR	STAGGS
69	MELINDA LEE	HEAD
69	PATRICIA ANDERSON	MORRISON
69	PATRICIA KATHLEEN KELLY	BROGAN
69	PATRICIA LARSON	GARSIDE
69	PATRICIA WALSH	RODRIGUES
69	PENNY BLAIR	ROGERS
69	ROSALIE WIESEHAHN	SHEVELAND
69	SANDRA BOWMAN	HASTINGS
69	SHARON BENNETT	MAST
69	SHEILA FITZGERALD	BATZ
69	SUSAN DETWEILER	PINCKARD
69	SUSAN HALL	WILLIAMS
69	TAMA	ADELMAN
69	TERRY CLARK	FOUSHEE
69	WILMYNA STUIT	GANDY
70	BILLIE COOEETTA	MEADOR
70	CAROL ANN	GLENN
70	CAROLYN FACCIANO	MACOMBER
70	CATHERINE WAIDTLOW	DUNNING
70	CHERYL HUTTON	PREBULA
70	CHRISTINE LITTLE	JACKSON
70	CONSTANCE HERBERT	SELBY
70	CYNTHIA CLARK	ARSHAD
70	DAIDRE FOOTE	WEST
70	DAPHNE SUZETTE	BEISEL
70	DEBORA JEAN CLARK	GAMBA
70	DEBORAH MEYER	JOHNSTON
70	DONNA	ROSE
70	DONNA DAKE METCALF	BALL
70	MARIETTA HARMON	SMITH
70	JANET ANN	CLEAVES
70	JANICE GREENWOOD	MUELLER
70	JANIE PAYNE	JOHANSEN
70	KATHLEEN COGAN	BEIERSCHMITT
70	KATHLEEN JONES	WILLIAMS
70	KATHLEEN MORTON	BURNS
70	MARTHA KATHLEEN BACA	KLEIN
70	KRIS VALETA PILLOW	FARWELL
70	KRISTINE SMITH	ROSENBERG
70	LINDA AHLIN	SULPRIZIO
70	LINDA GREENWOOD	SNODGRASS
70	MELANIE GAYLE	OBLENDER, MD
70	NANCY MILLER	O'BRIEN
70	NANCY RAPP	BELL
70	PAMELA GILL	LAM
70	PATRICIA OWENS	NOSSEN
70	PATRICCA SPARROWE	GAHAGAN
70	PATRICIA STEPHENS	BRENNEMAN
70	RAMONA RAE	CLARK
70	ROBIN WULFERT	ROGERS
70	SHARON LYNN KEMP	KILWEIN
70	SHERREY ROFF	WILLIAMS
70	SHIRELY ANN	PETERS
70	VICKY SURDEZ	FLICKINGER
70	VIRGINIA JEAN KRAMER	MORTH
70	VIVIAN KENNEDY	BRAILOFF
71	ANNE TEMPLIN	LYONS
71	ANNE VELS	PIERCE
71	BEVERLEY JANE DONNELL	SELIVANOV
71	BARBARA DAVIS	TAMBLIN
71	BARBARA MAC INTYRE	PALMER
71	BRENDA JONES	JOYNER
71	CHRISTINE KENNAN	FROELICH
71	CHRISTINE KIRKMAN	BLOODWORTH
71	CHRISTINE HAAXMA	NEWMAN
71	DAMARS ROCHELLE	DENNIS
71	DEANNA LYNN	BAIRD
71	DEBORAH KING	MARTINEZ
71	DEBORAH PRATER	GODINE
71	DIANE TROWER	SALGADO
71	DOLORES PLOTT	CORNETT
71	ELISA LOUGHMAN	FRANKE-JUKES
71	GLENNA OLDFIELD	MARTIN
71	JACQUELNE SULLIVAN	MCGINNIS
71	JOAN GREENWOOD	JOHNSON
71	JUDY WALTERS	BARNES
71	KAREN SPARKS	GNASS
71	KATHERINE NELLE NEIGHBOR	ALONZO
71	KATHLEEN FAGGART	LECHMAN
71	KATHLEEN FOUNCE	HALVIG
71	KRISTINA LUCICH	SANTOS
71	KRISTYN WITTE	WILSON
71	LAUREEN CARDOZA	SCHROEDER
71	LAUREL BURGESS	MURRAY
71	LEA NEUERBURG	MASON
71	LESLIE MC QUEEN	HOFFLER
71	LINDA JOYCE WOODY	WOOD
71	LINDA JOHNSTON	MOYLE
71	MAMIE GORDON	MOSSMAN
71	MARCIA BECKETT	RATTERREE
71	MARY LOUISE	SAYLOR
71	MARY LYNNE	KIESLING
71	MELVA ELAYNE WRIGHT	POWELL
71	PATRICIA BUENAVENTURA	CARLEY
71	ROBIN EDWARDS	MAXEY
71	SANDRA PARKER	YOUNG
71	SHIRLEY ANN	SPINK
71	TWILA BROEKEMIER	ALEXANDER
71	VICTORIA SOTO	ENDO
72	ALYS MARIE	MAINHART
72	ANGELA JANSSEN	FIELDER
72	ANNE L'AMOUREAUX	MAHER
72	BESSIE PARKER	FAHEY
72	BETHANY FREEMAN	GAMELIN
72	CECILLE	GARCIA
72	CLARIE ESPELAND	COUCH
72	CLAUDIA CHAFFIN	ANCONA
72	DEBRA CARTER	JACOBS
72	DIANA GREY	ALBRITTON
72	GAIL MIRANDA	WALKER
72	HELAH BETH ALDEMAN	BLUMHAGEN
72	HOLLY KAY	KRAMARSIC
72	JACQUELINE SOLGA	PHILLIPS
72	JACQUELINE THWAITS	MCCLURE
72	JANICE STRACNER	MC KINNEY
72	JEAN JONES	HIGGINS
72	JOAN PEDERSEN	CARR
72	KAREN JEANNE	LEWIS-MILLER
72	KATHLEEN LAURA	CHAPMAN
72	KATHLEEN MARIE	WALSH
72	KATHY JACOBSEN	RUSSO
72	LINDA GRAPES	GRAHMS
72	LUCINDA WYNANT	BEYER
72	MARGARET CASAREZ	SALLOMI
72	MARILYN JOAN	RIGGS
72	MARY ELIZABETH	AMBROSE
72	MAUREEN CROSSMAN	LUNDBOM
72	NANCY HARWOOD	PIERCE
72	NEDA BYLSMA	ANDERSON
72	PATRICIA BROWN	CONEY
72	PATTY HITCOCK	ALDRICH
72	PAULA GISI	ABRAHAM
72	REBECCA BUCHHOLZ	DAVIDSON

Year	First Name	Last Name
72	ROXANNE	CORLEY
72	RUTH VELDSTRA	PONSFORD
72	SANDRA DOAN	ROHLFING
72	SANDRA DUCHAINE	REIN
72	SHERYL SEARS	SWAN
72	SUSAN MARIE	CUNNINGHAM
72	SUSAN VERMEULEN	JAMISON
72	SUSAN WHITE	ELIAS
72	SUZANNE MICHA	SOMMER
72	THERESA KATHLEEN	SMELTZER
73	BARBARA SHEERAN	SMITH
73	BETTY JANE	COOK
73	CAROL	UNDERWOOD
73	CATHERINE GILL	DAVIS
73	CATHERINE HALEY	MC COOL
73	CHARLENE ALBRO	TAYLOR
73	CLARICE BROOKS	BRIDGES
73	CLARISSA BONNIE	FLIPPIN
73	CORAL REAVES	MATICH
73	CYNTHIA DICK	THOMASSON
73	CYNTHA JORGENSEN	WOODBURY
73	DEBORAH LYNN	LANNOM
73	DEBORAH REID	HORN
73	DEBORAH SUE	BRADEN
73	DEBORAH SUSAN	LARSON
73	DONALD ARTHUR	MORGAN
73	EILEEN FRANCES	HOFFMAN
73	ELIZABETH PEARSON	WELLMAN
73	GAIL SCHNEIDER	FREDERICK
73	HEIDI JANSSEN	RENTZ
73	IRENE DAVIDSON	THOMAS
73	JACALYN SCHNEIDER	BROOKS
73	JANE WANDA	CARLSON
73	JANICE FINK SMITH	JAMAGATA
73	JEANNE LOUISE	HILL
73	JOAN BROOKS	ALHINO
73	JOAN CONCANNON	ENCARNACION
73	JO MICHAEL BEARD	DUKE
73	JOSEPHINE BALESTRIERI	FRANCK
73	KATHERINE	SMITH
73	KATHY TYSINGER	TOMLIN
73	KRISTIN	WEAVER
73	LINDA ANN	MORGAN
73	LINDA DEVINE	FOWLER
73	LINDA GORE	THOMAS
73	MARGARET FRIEDRICH	EVANS
73	MARY BAXTER	HOWARD
73	MARY JO WRIGHT	BOYLON
73	MARY WARD	GALLINA
73	MAUREEN	WILLIAMS
73	NANCY HASKINS	MCCLURE
73	PAMELA BROWN	JENKINS
73	PATRICIA KOPACHE	FITCH
73	PATRICIA MERENDA	FORG
73	PATRICIA PRUEHER	LANNING
73	ROBIN GROSS	GARRETT
73	RUTH HOLLAND	JONES
73	SHARON VAUGHAN	ELLIS
72	SHIRELY HUFFMAN	SCHNEIDER
73	SUSAN KENDALL	JONES
73	SUSAN MOSCARELLI MARTIN	CATLING
73	TEREAL MC GINLEY	DAMMEL
73	TERESE MAYES	REVAK
73	VALERIE TOSTE	OBRIEN
73	VULA ROED	GUTMAN
74	AMY STROSINA	ANDERSON
74	ANDREA LEE	LANGLEY
74	AUDREY WELCH	MATHESON
74	BARBARA UCOVICH	HETTELSATER
74	BONNIE BUFORD	CASHER
74	CAROLYN LEE	DORSEY
74	CAROLYN MC NAMARA	BRADON
74	CHRISTINE ANN	WESTCOTT
74	CHRISTINE COULSON	BECKET
74	DEBORAH FULFORD	JONES
74	DEBORAH SUE	BUGEL
74	DIANNA CHAN	LOY
74	DIANE VETTER	MCCLENATHAN
74	DONNA YVONNE	COLLINS
74	ELIZABETH ANN	MARTIN
74	GALE MARIE CARLI	SIMMONS
74	ILENE MERLE	CRAFT
74	JANICE CLAUDIA	WARNECKE
74	JEFFREY WILLIAM	PURTLE
74	JOAN MARIE	FARWELL
74	KAROLYN RIBBLE	COMES
74	KATHLEEN ANN	SCHUPRACH
74	KATHLEEN JOAN	MAYER
74	KATHLYN JO	BENOIT
74	KAYE HARKER	HANSEN
74	LAYNE	KRAMER
74	LOYOLA RAMONA	SCHULER
74	LYNN OLSON	MERRITT
74	LYNN PADRNOS	WORHAM
74	MARCIE FOSTER	RODRIGUEZ
74	MARIAN BRIDGES	SHULL
74	MARILYN	CALLEGARI
74	MARILYN GLARE	HEDQUIST
74	MARY LEONA	PHELAN
74	NORMA BOLLA	FELLNER
74	PEGGY LYNN	SHREVE
74	SUSAN TANNER	DRABIN
74	TENA LORRAINE	AUSTIN
74	TERI VANCE	BEROER
74	WENDY ARONSEN	CORR
74	YOLANDA IZQUIERDO	PRIZE
75	ALICIA SANTOS	HUGHES
75	ANN MARIE DeCOSTA	GRIFFIN
75	ANN THORNALLY	BRURUD
75	BARBARA GOODMAN	UHRIE
75	BARBARA J ANE	SHELTON
75	BEVERLY BAILEY	BARTON
75	BRENDA VIDALE	BARBER
75	CELESTE MARIE	SCHREIBER
75	CHARELE VERONICA	REILLY
76	CHERYL ANN	PRINCE
75	CHERYL ELLEN	WRAA
75	CHRISTINE DONAHUE	HAMRICK
75	CHRISTY DODGE	SHAW
75	DEANNA LORRIE	MANN
75	DESORAH ANNE	PETERS
75	DENISE ARLEEN	CHANEY
75	DEVON FRANCES	ROETH
75	DONALD THOMAS	MANCUSO
75	ELIZABETH ANN	HAGEN
75	ELIZABETH MILLER	FRECHETTE
75	FATH MARIE	SANTOS
75	JACQUELINE ANN	SHERROW
75	JEAN	ZIMMERMAN
75	JOANNE RUTLAND	MOODY
75	JUDITH ANN	BERGE
75	KATHLEEN ROCK	STALLWORTH
75	LARRY ALLEN	MALATO
75	LAURA ANN	SERGEANT
75	LORRANE KATHLEEN	BOURNE
75	MARISA CRISTINA	HERNANDEZ
75	MARTHA ANN	STEWERT
75	MAUREEN CECILE	WOLLARD
75	MAXINE DONER	SHEDD
75	MICHELLE LEGGINS	TANTARELLI
75	NANCY ANN	BURNETTE
75	RICCI LYNN RIMPAU	CLELAND
75	SHARMEL THOMPSON	DUNN
75	SHEILA HARTMAN	FRIES
75	STELLA TATSUYO	MARUBAYASHI
75	SUE ANN	TARLETON
75	TERESA FAUSNAUGHT	CAIN

75	ZOANNE MYRA	HYLAND	76	GAIL KIMIKO DATE	YAMAMOTO	76	MARSHA BELSKY	YOUSEF
			76	GERALDINE FORGNONI	VERVERS	76	MAYUMI NISHI	TANIMURA
76	ANITA LOUISE MART	GORDON	76	JANICE SHAFFER	HORTON	76	MERRI BETH BLAKE	MARX
76	ARLENE WONG	LUM	76	JOHN CONRAD	DEXHEIMER	76	MICHELE DIANNE	HURD
76	AVA DENISE BOWDEN	GOINS	76	JOYCE YUKIYE	ENDO	76	NANCY TOBIN	SEARLE
76	BARBARA SINTON	TRIMBUR	76	JUDITH MURRAY ANDERSON	GOTTLIEB	76	NIKOLET BOSKI	SHELTON
76	BERNADETTE REYNOSO	LIGHTFOOT	76	JUDY ANN ROSA	CHESSAR	76	PAMELA ANN MANDT	REILLEY
76	BERYL ANN	SHAW	76	KAREN SCHRODER	LEWIS	76	PATRICIA ROSINE	KOVALCHECK
76	CASSANDRA FAY	MC DOWELL	76	KATHLEEN KIRROS	BACA	76	PENNY WIEGERS	MORRIS
76	CHARIS YOUNG	SUBIL	76	KATHY KOFNOVEC	CORZINE	76	PETER JULIO	GUZMAN
76	CHRISTINE	MUDGE	76	KIMBERLY HUEBNER	BERGGREN	76	RITA MAE	SHAFFER
76	CLAUDIA HEINEMANN	WALKER	76	LAUREL BENGARD	PLASKETT	76	ROSALINDA CAMARILLO	TOVAR
76	CONSTANCE SARAH	PRESENT	76	LINETTE REILLY	HAMIL	76	SHARON TOLTON	SCOLNICK
76	DANIELLE SNEAHAN	ANGELI	76	LORI WALLECK	RYAN	76	SHERRY SWETNMAN	WEBBER
76	DAVID KEVIN	SMITH	76	MARGARET MOORE	WALDHAUS	76	STEPHANIE SAUER	CIOTTI
76	DEBRA	LENT	76	MARGARET YOU TSING	CHANG	76	STEVEN ROBERT	FERNALD
76	DENISE DAWSON	COSTA	76	MARILYN ELAINE	STEWART	76	SUZANNE WELCH	KINZLI
76	DONNA CATHERINE	REARDON	76	MARJORIE ANN	JORDAN	76	TELOA SEGREST	SIMMONS
76	DORIS BOLOMEY	IRONS	76	MARJORIE EILEEN	PEDROZA			

KFSN Graduates Who Led or Were "Firsts" to Help Define Kaiser Permanente

Over the 70+ year history of the KFSN, many graduates assumed leadership roles within Kaiser Permanente. Some graduates became instructors at the school; many became leaders in administrative and management positions – leading nursing staff and service units – as directors, managers, and supervisors. Although it is not possible to identify all KFSN graduates who held leadership roles within Kaiser Permanente, a few are notable in that they held top administrative positions or they were the "first" in positions that helped define the organization.

- DORRIS FACEY LOVRIN, Class of 50 — After graduating from the first class, she opened the new San Francisco Hospital as its first nurse. She continued working there for over 60 years in the Emergency Department, teaching CPR in the last few years until she finally retired at 84 years old.

- CLAIR O'SULLIVAN LISKER, Class of '51A — Instructor and associate director at the school; became the chief nursing officer at the Oakland Hospital. Retired after 43 years having touched the lives of all KFSN graduates.

- JESSIE HEAD CUNNINGHAM, Class of '54 — First African American nurse supervisor at the Oakland Hospital. Retired after 45 years.

- LA VERNE OYARZO, Class of '54 — TPMG's first medical nurse practitioner while heading up Oakland's Multiphasic Health Assessment Program.

- PHYLLIS PLANT MORONEY, Class of '57A — TPMG's first pediatric nurse practitioner at the Oakland Clinic.

- GRETCHEN MUELLER SEIFERT, Class of '59 — Medical Center Administrator at both Martinez and Walnut Creek; became Program Office Vice President for Quality. First nurse in a top executive position. Retired after 36 years.

- DELORAS PLAKE JONES, Class of '63 — Chief nursing officer at the San Francisco Hospital; became KP's first California and health system chief nursing executive. Retired after 37 years.

- LINDA TAYLOR, Class of '64 — Following leadership positions at the Oakland Medical Offices, joined Regional Labor Relations as the first to represent the nursing voice in Labor Relations. Retired after 38 years.

- DEANA CARTER MEDINAS, Class of '66 — Medical Group Administrator at the Hayward Medical Offices. Retired after 47 years.

- MARY HEALY THODE, Class of '66 — Regional Administrator of Northern California, then President of Kaiser Foundation Health Plan and Hospitals, Northern California Region. Shattered KP's glass ceiling.

Endnotes

PROLOGUE

1   Personal communication of Dr. Ted Eytan, former medical director for The Kaiser Permanente Center for Total Health in Washington, D.C., with Deloras Plake Jones, May 4, 2017.

2   Jim D'Alfonso, DNP, RN, Ph.D.(h), NEA-BC, FNAP, Deloras Jones, MSN, RN, and Terri Moss, BA, "Kaiser's School of Nursing: A 70-Year Legacy of Disruptive Innovation," *Nursing Administration Quarterly*, January/March 2018, p. 35.

CHAPTER 1

1   Steve Gilford interview of Elizabeth Runyen Baeker, Colfax, California, September 24, 1993. Transcripts on file at the Kaiser Permanente Archives, Oakland, California.

2   Kaiser Permanente archives; interview with Dr. Sidney Garfield, Oakland, California, 1974.

3   "Final Report of the Committee on the Costs of Medical Care," *New England Journal of Medicine*, December 1, 1932; p. 996.

4   Joseph S. Ross, "The Committee on the Cost of Medical Care and the History of Health Insurance in the US," *The Einstein Quarterly Journal of Biology & Medicine*, 2002, p. 129.

5   Steve Gilford interview of Cecil Cutting, 1974. Transcript on file at the Kaiser Permanente Archives, Oakland, California. Steve Gilford interviews of Geraldine Searcy and Rae Englemann, Oakland, California, August 1992. Notes are in interviewer's collection, Petaluma, California.

6   Kaiser Permanente archives; interview with Dr. Sidney Garfield, Oakland, California, September 4, 1974.

7   Ibid.

8   Tom Debley, *The Story of Dr. Sidney Garfield: The Visionary Who Turned Sick Care into Health Care*, The Permanente Press, 2009, p. 33.

9   Ibid.

10   Kaiser Permanente Archives; interview with Cecil Cutting, Oakland, California.

11   Tom Debley, *The Story of Dr. Sidney Garfield: The Visionary Who Turned Sick Care into Health Care*, The Permanente Press, 2009, p. 37.

12   Moss Avenue later would be renamed MacArthur Boulevard to honor Gen. Douglas MacArthur.

13   Steve Gilford interview of Geraldine Searcy, RN, Oakland, California, August 1992. Notes are in interviewer's collection, Petaluma, California.

14   John G. Smillie, *Can Physicians Manage the Quality and Costs of Health Care?: The Story of the Permanente Medical Group*, McGraw-Hill, 1991, p. 42.

15   Steve Gilford interview of Rae Englemann, Oakland, California, August 1992. Notes are in interviewer's collection, Petaluma, California.

16   Steve Gifford and Tom Debley interview of Harriet Stewart, Oakland, California, June 2002. Transcript on file at the Kaiser Permanente Archives, Oakland, California.

CHAPTER 2

1   Fore 'N' Aft magazine, Henry Kaiser's address at the dedication of the Fabiola Hospital, August 1942.

2   Sidney Garfield, "2nd Annual Report of the Permanente Foundation Hospital," *Permanente Foundation Medical Bulletin*, January 1945, p. 33.

3   The name of the Permanente School of Nursing would be changed in 1953 to the Kaiser Foundation School of Nursing.

4   In the hysteria following the surprise Japanese attack on the U.S. forces in Pearl Harbor on Dec. 7, 1941, President Roosevelt issued Executive Order 9066, giving the military broad powers to ban any citizen deemed potentially dangerous from a 50- to 60-mile-wide coastal strip from Washington state to California, extending inland into southern Arizona. It also authorized transporting these citizens, primarily Japanese Americans, to 10 military-controlled camps in remote areas of Arizona, California, Idaho, Oregon, Utah and Wyoming; 110,000 people were confined for the duration of the war.

5 Sidney Garfield, *The Permanente Bulletin*, 1945; Kaiser Permanente Archives, Oakland, California.

6 John G. Smillie, *Can Physicians Manage the Quality and Costs of Health Care?: The Story of the Permanente Medical Group*, McGraw-Hill, 1991, p. 140.

7 Albert P. Heiner, *Henry J. Kaiser: Western Colossus*, Halo Books, 1991, p. 91.

8 https://kpnursing.org/_NCAL/professionaldevelopment/alumni/history.html, accessed February 4, 2020.

9 Oral History of Avram Yedidia, University of California Bancroft Library, Regional Oral History Office, 1982.

10 There were no wards in the hospital, only two-bed rooms.

11 All quotes from nursing school alumni come either from questionnaires sent to each of them or from interviews conducted by Steve Gilford between May 2017 and October 2019. More than 700 pages of transcripts of these interviews, as well as the hundreds of questionnaires, are located at the Kaiser Permanente Archives, Oakland, California.

12 Steve Gilford interview of Francine Weir Ammerman, Oakland, California, August 29, 2017. Transcript on file at the Kaiser Permanente Archives, Oakland, California.

13 Clair Lisker, "A Voice for Nursing Education, Kaiser Permanente, 1948–1991," interview conducted by Judith Dunnings in 2002, Regional Oral History Office, The Bancroft Library, University of California, Berkeley, 2002, p. 34.

14 Student Handbook, 1948 Permanente School of Nursing.

15 Kaiser Permanente Archives, Henry J. Kaiser, Remarks at the Commencement Exercises, Permanente School of Nursing, August 25, 1950.

16 Steve Gilford interview of William Soule, Oakland, California, October 21, 1991. Notes in interviewer's collection, Petaluma, California.

17 "Iron nurse Dorothea Daniels had a soft spot for nursing students," https://about.kaiserpermanente.org/our-story/our-history/iron-nurse-dorothea-daniels-had-a-soft-spot-for-nursing-students, accessed February 5, 2020.

18 Dorothea Daniels, "What Ninety Girls Like to Do in Their Spare Time," *American Journal of Nursing*, November 1940, p. 1248.

19 Steve Gilford interview of James Vohs, Oakland, California, September 15, 2017. Transcript on file at the Kaiser Permanente Archives, Oakland, California.

20 John G. Smillie, *Can Physicians Manage the Quality and Costs of Health Care?: The Story of the Permanente Medical Group*, McGraw-Hill, 1991, p. 107.

21 Steve Gilford interview of Janice Klein, Oakland, California, June 12, 2017. Transcript on file at the Kaiser Permanente Archives, Oakland, California.

22 Steve Gilford interview of Ethel O'Donnell Morgan, Oakland, California, December 20, 2017. Transcript on file at the Kaiser Permanente Archives, Oakland, California.

23 Steve Gilford interview of Naomi Eiko Tanikawa, Oakland, California, November 10, 2017. Transcript on file at the Kaiser Permanente Archives, Oakland, California.

24 Steve Gilford interview of Francine Weir Ammerman, Oakland, California, November 29, 2017. Transcript on file at the Kaiser Permanente Archives, Oakland, California.

25 Steve Gilford interview of Ethel O'Donnell Morgan, Oakland, California, December 20, 2017. Transcript on file at the Kaiser Permanente Archives, Oakland, California.

26 Steve Gilford interview of Francine Weir Ammerman, Oakland, California, August 29, 2017. Transcript on file at the Kaiser Permanente Archives, Oakland, California.

27 Steve Gilford interview of Clair O'Sullivan Lisker, Oakland, California, July 25, 1992. Notes in interviewer's collection, Petaluma, California.

28 Ibid.

29 Steve Gilford interview of Francine Weir Ammerman, Oakland, California, August 29, 2017. Transcript on file at the Kaiser Permanente Archives, Oakland, California.

30 Steve Gilford interview of Clair O'Sullivan Lisker, Oakland, California, January 31, 2018. Transcript on file at the Kaiser Permanente Archives, Oakland, California.

31 Steve Gilford interview of Clair O'Sullivan Lisker, Oakland, California, January 21, 1992. Notes in interviewer's collection, Petaluma, California.

32 Steve Gilford interview of Lesley Meriwether, Oakland, California, November 22, 2017. Transcript on file at the Kaiser Permanente Archives, Oakland, California.

33 Steve Gilford interview of Clair O'Sullivan Lisker, Oakland, California, January 3, 2018. Transcript on file at the Kaiser Permanente Archives, Oakland, California.

34 Steve Gilford interview of Francine Weir Ammerman, Oakland, California, August 29, 2017. Transcript on file at the Kaiser Permanente Archives, Oakland, California.

35 Steve Gilford interview of Bea Rudney, Oakland, California, August 15, 2017. Transcript on file at the Kaiser Permanente Archives, Oakland, California.

36 Steve Gilford interview of Sharon Scolnick, Oakland, California, October 3, 2019. Transcript on file at the Kaiser Permanente Archives, Oakland, California.

37 Steve Gilford interview of Bea Rudney, Oakland, California, August 15, 2017. Transcript on file at the Kaiser Permanente Archives, Oakland, California.

38 Steve Gilford interview of Marion Yeaw, Oakland, California, May 18, 2017. Transcript on file at the Kaiser Permanente Archives, Oakland, California.

39 "Iron nurse Dorothea Daniels had a soft spot for nursing students," https://about.kaiserpermanente.org/our-story/our-history/iron-nurse-dorothea-daniels-had-a-soft-spot-for-nursing-students, accessed February 5, 2020.

CHAPTER 3

1 John G. Smillie, *Can Physicians Manage the Quality and Costs of Health Care?: The Story of the Permanente Medical Group*, McGraw-Hill, 1991, p. 71.

2 The Permanente Medical Group referred only to the Northern California medical group. As Kaiser Permanente expanded to other parts of the country, the medical groups took on distinctive titles, e.g., Southern California Permanente Medical Group.

3 Margretta M. Styles, *On Nursing: Toward a New Endowment*, Mosby Inc., 1982, p. 160.

4 California Medical Association: H. Gordon MacLean, president-elect, *California Medicine*, 1950, p. 470, https://eurekamag.com/research/051/910/051910243.php, accessed February 4, 2020.

5 Steve Gilford telephone conversation with Clifford Keene, April 12, 1995. Notes in interviewer's collection, Petaluma, California.

6 Steve Gilford interview of Bea Rudney, Oakland, California, August 15, 2017. Transcript on file at the Kaiser Permanente Archives, Oakland, California.

7 Steve Gilford interview of Janice Price Klein, Oakland, California, June 12, 2017. Transcript on file at the Kaiser Permanente Archives, Oakland, California.

8 Steve Gilford interview of Nancy Horie Suda, Oakland, California, June 5, 2017. Transcript on file at the Kaiser Permanente Archives, Oakland, California.

9 Steve Gilford interview of Ethel O'Donnell Morgan, Oakland, California, December 20, 2017. Transcript on file at the Kaiser Permanente Archives, Oakland, California.

10 Steve Gilford interview of Francine Weir Ammerman, Oakland, California, August 9, 2017. Transcript on file at the Kaiser Permanente Archives, Oakland, California.

11 Steve Gilford interview of Helen Harrison Robinson, Oakland, California, September 6, 2017. Transcript on file at the Kaiser Permanente Archives, Oakland, California.

12 Ibid.

13 Steve Gilford interview of Phyllis Plant Moroney, Oakland, California, September 20, 2017. Transcript on file at the Kaiser Permanente Archives, Oakland, California.

14 Steve Gilford interview of Grace Oshita Miyamoto, Oakland, California, November 14, 2017. Transcript on file at the Kaiser Permanente Archives, Oakland, California.

15 Ibid.

16 Ibid.

17 Ibid.

18 Ibid.

19 Steve Gilford interview of Rebecca Schoenthal Calloway, Oakland, California, January 22, 2018. Transcript on file at the Kaiser Permanente Archives, Oakland, California.

20 Steve Gilford interview of Lynn DeForest Robie, Oakland, California, September 8, 2017. Transcript on file at the Kaiser Permanente Archives, Oakland, California.

21 Steve Gilford interview of Nelle Neighbor Alonzo, Oakland, California, October 2, 2017. Transcript on file at the Kaiser Permanente Archives, Oakland, California.

22 Steve Gilford interview of Marion Yeaw, Oakland, California, June 18, 2017. Transcript on file at the Kaiser Permanente Archives, Oakland, California.

23 Steve Gilford interview of Juliette Whitfield Powell, Oakland, California, December 2, 2017. Transcript on file at the Kaiser Permanente Archives, Oakland, California.

24 John G. Smillie, *Can Physicians Manage the Quality and Costs of Health Care?: The Story of the Permanente Medical Group*, McGraw-Hill, 1991, p. 42.

25 Steve Gilford interview of Clair O'Sullivan Lisker, Oakland, California, January 31, 2018. Transcript on file at the Kaiser Permanente Archives, Oakland, California.

26 Steve Gilford interview of Janice Price Klein, Oakland, California, June 12, 2017. Transcript on file at the Kaiser Permanente Archives, Oakland, California.

27 Steve Gilford interview of Grace Oshita Miyamoto, Oakland, California, November 14, 2017. Transcript on file at the Kaiser Permanente Archives, Oakland, California.

28 Steve Gilford interview of Marion Yeaw, Oakland, California, June 18, 2017. Transcript on file at the Kaiser Permanente Archives, Oakland, California.

29 Ibid.

30 Ibid.

31 Ibid.

32 Ibid.

33 Steve Gilford interview of Phyllis Plant Moroney, Oakland, California, September 20, 2017. Transcript on file at the Kaiser Permanente Archives, Oakland, California.

34 Steve Gilford interview of Clair O'Sullivan Lisker, Oakland, California, January 31, 2018. Transcript on file at the Kaiser Permanente Archives, Oakland, California.

35 Steve Gilford interview of Lynn DeForest Robie, Oakland, California, September 8, 2017. Transcript on file at the Kaiser Permanente Archives, Oakland, California.

36 Steve Gilford interview of Jean Berg Meddaugh, Oakland, California, November 16, 2017. Transcript on file at the Kaiser Permanente Archives, Oakland, California.

37 Ibid.

38 Steve Gilford interview of Marilyn Nystrom Aiken, Oakland, California, November 29, 2017. Transcript on file at the Kaiser Permanente Archives, Oakland, California.

39 Ibid.

40 Steve Gilford interview of Sylvia Barnes Bertram, Oakland, California, June 2, 2017. Transcript on file at the Kaiser Permanente Archives, Oakland, California.

41 Steve Gilford interview of Marilyn Nystrom Aiken, Oakland, California, November 29, 2017. Transcript on file at the Kaiser Permanente Archives, Oakland, California.

42 Ibid.

43 Steve Gilford interview of Ron Bachman, MD, Oakland, California, August 14, 2017. Transcript on file at the Kaiser Permanente Archives, Oakland, California.

44 Ibid.

45 "The Drawsheet," October 1953, Kaiser Permanente Archives.

46 John G. Smillie, *Can Physicians Manage the Quality and Costs of Health Care?: The Story of the Permanente Medical Group*, McGraw-Hill, 1991, p. 93.

CHAPTER 4

1 Steve Gilford interview of Bea Rudney, Oakland, California, August 15, 2017. Transcript on file at the Kaiser Permanente Archives, Oakland, California.

2 Steve Gilford interview of Lesley Meriwether, Oakland, California, August 22, 2017. Transcript on file at the Kaiser Permanente Archives, Oakland, California.

3 Ibid.

4 Ibid.

5 Steve Gilford interview of Gretchen Mueller Seifert, Oakland, California, August 16, 2017. Transcript on file at the Kaiser Permanente Archives, Oakland, California.

6 Steve Gilford interview of Elizabeth Ann Miller Moore, Oakland, California, August 15, 2017. Transcript on file at the Kaiser Permanente Archives, Oakland, California.

7 Ruth Tolman, *The Nurse's Guide to Beauty, Charm, Poise*, Milady Publishing Corp., 1963.

8 Steve Gilford interview of Elizabeth Ann Miller Moore, Oakland, California, January 22, 2018. Transcript on file at the Kaiser Permanente Archives, Oakland, California.

9 Steve Gilford interview of Rebecca Schoenthal Calloway, Oakland, California, January 22, 2018. Transcript on file at the Kaiser Permanente Archives, Oakland, California.

10 Steve Gilford interview with Kristin Weaver, Oakland, California, September 11, 2019. Transcript on file at the Kaiser Permanente Archives, Oakland, California.

11 Steve Gilford conversation with Deloras Plake Jones, Oakland, California, April 28, 2019.

12 Dorothea Daniels, "What Ninety Girls Like to do in Their Spare Time," *American Journal of Nursing*, November 1940, p. 1248.

13 Steve Gilford interview of Lynn DeForest Robie, Oakland, California, September 8, 2017. Transcript on file at the Kaiser Permanente Archives, Oakland, California.

14 Steve Gilford interview of Elizabeth Ann Miller Moore, Oakland, California, August 15, 2017. Transcript on file at the Kaiser Permanente Archives, Oakland, California.

15 Steve Gilford interview of Mary Louise Mott, Oakland, California, September 18, 2017. Transcript on file at the Kaiser Permanente Archives, Oakland, California.

16 Nurse Training Act of 1964, Public Law 88-581, September 4, 1964, www.govinfo.gov/content/pkg/STATUTE-78/pdf/STATUTE-78-Pg908-2.pdf#page=6; Eric.ed.gov/fulltext/ED028240pdf accessed February 12, 2020.

17 Kaiser Permanente newsletter, December 9, 1968. On file at the Kaiser Permanente Archives, Oakland, California.

18 Undated mimeo sheet. On file at the Kaiser Permanente Archives, Oakland, California.

19 Steve Gilford interview of Elizabeth Ann Miller Moore, Oakland, California, September 8, 2017. Transcript on file at the Kaiser Permanente Archives, Oakland, California.

20 Steve Gilford interview of Gail Sinquefeld, Oakland, California, August 25, 2017. Transcript on file at the Kaiser Permanente Archives, Oakland, California.

21 Steve Gilford interview of Cynthia Reed, Oakland, California, August 31, 2017. Transcript on file at the Kaiser Permanente Archives, Oakland, California.

22 Steve Gilford interview of Grace Oshita Miyamoto, Oakland, California, November 14, 2017. Transcript on file at the Kaiser Permanente Archives, Oakland, California.

23 Steve Gilford interview of Cynthia Reed, Oakland, California, August 31, 2017. Transcript on file at the Kaiser Permanente Archives, Oakland, California.

24 Steve Gilford interview of Grace Oshita Miyamoto, Oakland, California, November 14, 2017. Transcript on file at the Kaiser Permanente Archives, Oakland, California.

25 Steve Gilford interview of Clair O'Sullivan Lisker, Oakland, California, January 31, 2018. Transcript on file at the Kaiser Permanente Archives, Oakland, California.

26 Ibid.

27 Steve Gilford interview of Jeff Purtle, Oakland, California, January 17, 2018. Transcript on file at the Kaiser Permanente Archives, Oakland, California.

28 Starting in 1969, entering classes were issued the school's new uniform, a yellow and white shift-style Dacron outfit with a simplified apron, a perma-starched cap and an all-weather coat of either blue or gold.

29 Steve Gilford interview of Jeff Purtle, Oakland, California, January 17, 2018. Transcript on file at the Kaiser Permanente Archives, Oakland, California.

30 Steve Gilford interview of Bea Rudney, Oakland, California, August 15, 2017. Transcript on file at the Kaiser Permanente Archives, Oakland, California.

31 Steve Gilford interview of Jeff Purtle, Oakland, California, January 17, 2018. Transcript on file at the Kaiser Permanente Archives, Oakland, California.

32 Steve Gilford interview of Francine Weir Ammerman, Oakland, California, November 20, 2017. Transcript on file at the Kaiser Permanente Archives, Oakland, California.

33 Steve Gilford interview of Clair O'Sullivan Lisker, Oakland, California, January 31, 2018. Transcript on file at the Kaiser Permanente Archives, Oakland, California.

34 Steve Gilford interview of Cynthia Reed, Oakland, California, August 22, 2017. Transcript on file at the Kaiser Permanente Archives, Oakland, California.

35 Steve Gilford interview of Mary Ann Healy Thode, Oakland, California, September 26, 2018. Transcript on file at the Kaiser Permanente Archives, Oakland, California.

36 Steve Gilford interview of Lesley Meriwether, Oakland, California, August 22, 2017. Transcript on file at the Kaiser Permanente Archives, Oakland, California.

37 Steve Gilford interview of Mary Ann Healy Thode, Oakland, California, September 26, 2018. Transcript on file at the Kaiser Permanente Archives, Oakland, California.

38 Steve Gilford interview of Janice Price Klein, Oakland, California, June 12, 2017. Transcript on file at the Kaiser Permanente Archives, Oakland, California.

39 Steve Gilford interview of Jo Michael Beard Duke, Oakland, California, September 27, 2017. Transcript on file at the Kaiser Permanente Archives, Oakland, California.

40 Steve Gilford interview of Helen Harrison Robinson, Oakland, California, September 6, 2017. Transcript on file at the Kaiser Permanente Archives, Oakland, California.

41 California Board of Registered Nursing, www.rn.ca.gov, accessed February 10, 2020.

42 Steve Gilford interview of Nelle Neighbor Alonzo, Oakland, California, October 2, 2017. Transcript on file at the Kaiser Permanente Archives, Oakland, California.

43 Steve Gilford interview of Jeff Purtle, Oakland, California, January 17, 2018. Transcript on file at the Kaiser Permanente Archives, Oakland, California.

44 Steve Gilford interview of Juliette Whitfield Powell, Oakland, California, December 15, 2017. Transcript on file at the Kaiser Permanente Archives, Oakland, California.

CHAPTER 5

1 Clair Lisker, "A Voice for Nursing Education, Kaiser Permanente, 1948–1991," interview conducted by Judith Dunnings in 2002, Regional Oral History Office, The Bancroft Library, University of California, Berkeley, 2002.

2 John G. Smillie, *Can Physicians Manage the Quality and Costs of Health Care?: The Story of The Permanente Medical Group*, McGraw-Hill, Inc. 1991, p. 92.

3 Steve Gilford interview of Cynthia Reed, Oakland, California, August 3, 2017. Transcript on file at the Kaiser Permanente Archives, Oakland, California.

4 Minutes of the November 14, 1973, meeting of the Kaiser Foundation School of Nursing Board of Trustees. Notes on file in the offices of The Permanente Medical Group, Oakland, California.

5 Steve Gilford interview of Sharon Tolton Scolnick, Oakland, California, October 3, 2019. Transcript on file at the Kaiser Permanente Archives, Oakland, California.

6 Ibid.

7 Steve Gilford interview of James Vohs, Oakland, California, September 15, 2017. Transcript on file at the Kaiser Permanente Archives, Oakland.

8   John G. Smillie, *Can Physicians Manage the Quality and Costs of Health Care?: The Story of The Permanente Medical Group*, McGraw-Hill, Inc. 1991, p. 93.

CHAPTER 6

1   KFSN Alumni Association-provided information.

2   Kaiser Permanente Program for Alumni Graduation Dinner, June 11, 1976, Kaiser Permanente Archives, Oakland, California.

3   Teri Ann Allen, SCPMG ... *the First Fifty Years – History of the Southern California Kaiser Permanente Medical Group*, SCPMG, 2003, p. 81.

4   Steve Gilford interview of Phyllis Plant Moroney, Oakland, California, September 20, 2017. Transcript on file at the Kaiser Permanente Archives, Oakland, California.

5   Ibid.

6   Ibid.

7   California Assembly Bill No. 2629, July 17, 1984.

8   Personal communication of Geri Simmons, nursing education consultant, California Board of Registered Nursing, with Deloras Jones, regional nursing consultant, Northern California Kaiser Permanente Region, January 21, 1985.

9   Personal communication of Linda X. Fahey, leader for nurse practitioner practice, Southern California Permanente Medical Care Program, with Deloras Jones, regional nursing consultant, Northern California Kaiser Permanente Region, April 21, 1999.

10 Tom Debley, *The Story of Dr. Sidney Garfield: The Visionary Who Turned Sick Care into Health Care*, The Permanente Press, 2009, p. 101.

11 Steve Gilford interview of Phyllis Plant Moroney, Oakland, California, August 17, 2017. Notes are in interviewer's collection.

12 M. Yanover, D. Jones and M. Miller, "Perinatal Care of Low-Risk Mothers and Infants," *New England Journal of Medicine*, March 25, 1976, p. 702.

13 "Position Paper: Alternative in Maternity Care," *American Journal of Public Health*, March 1980, p. 14.

14 Personal communication of FAMCAP's physician co-leads, Dr. Mark Yanover and Dr. Michael Miller, with Deloras Plake Jones, 1980.

15 Alfred W. Brann, et al., "Criteria for Early Infant Discharge and Followup Evaluation," *Pediatrics*, March 1980, p. 651.

16 www.rn.ca.gov/pdfs/regulations/npr-b-20.pdf.

17 D. Jones and L. Close, "California Collaborative Model of Nursing Education: Building a Higher-Educated Nursing Workforce," *Nursing Economics*, November–December 2015, p. 335.

18 T. Bargagliotti, et al., "Joint Venture Arrangement for RN to BSN," *Nursing and Health Care*, September 1991, p. 380.

19 Personal communication of Debora Zachau with Deloras Jones, January 26, 2020, Oakland, California. In Jones' files.

20 Personal communication of Dorcas Walton with Deloras Jones, January 24, 2020, Oakland, California. In Jones' files.

21 https://about.kaiserpermanente.org/who-we-are/fast-facts.

22 KP Nursing Milestones: 1996–2016 used by permission of KP National Patient Care Services.

23 PPM image used by permission of KP National Patient Care Services.

24 KT. Waxman, J. D'Alfonso et al., "The AONE nurse executive competencies: 12 years later," *Nurse Leader*, April 2017, p. 120.

25 Daniel T. Linnen, Priscilla S. Javed and Jim D'Alfonso, "Ripe for Disruption? Adopting Nurse-Led Data Science and Artificial Intelligence to Predict and Reduce Hospital-Acquired Outcomes in the Learning Health System," *NAQ: Nursing Administration Quarterly*, July/September 2019, p. 246.

26 J. D'Alfonso and P.B. Winter, "A Systems Approach to Cultivate a Flourishing Nurse Workforce," *JCEN: The Journal of Continuing Education in Nursing*, June 2019, p. 248.

27 www.aacnnursing.org/Academic-Practice-Partnerships/Exemplary-Academic-Practice-Partnership-Award-Winners-and-Exemplars/Past-Award-Winners.

28 https://about.kaiserpermanente.org/our-story/our-care/kaiser-permanente-irvine-medical-center-achieves-magnet-recognit.

29 https://about.kaiserpermanente.org/our-story/our-care/kaiser-permanente-anaheim-medical-center-achieves-magnet-recogni.

30 Matthew D. McHugh, et al., "Achieving Kaiser Permanente Quality," *Health Care Management Review*, July–September 2016, p. 178.

31 J. D'Alfonso, D. Jones and T. Moss, "Kaiser's School of Nursing: A 70-Year Legacy of Disruptive Innovation," *NAQ: Nursing Administration Quarterly*, April/June 2018, p. 114.

32 J. D'Alfonso, et al., "Leading the Future We Envision: Nurturing a Culture of Innovation Across the Continuum of Care," *NAQ: Nursing Administration Quarterly*, January/March 2016, p. 68.

ABOUT THE EDITORS

Deloras Jones RN, MS

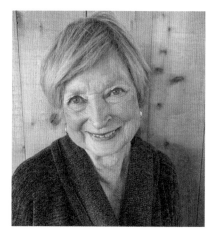

Deloras Jones RN, MS

Class of 1963 and Retired Health System Chief Nurse

Executive, Kaiser Permanente, Oakland, California

Deloras Jones retired from Kaiser Permanente in 2000 after a 37-year career with the organization – a career that began as a student at the Kaiser Foundation School of Nursing and ended as the organization's first system-wide Chief Nurse Executive. Upon her retirement, Kaiser Permanente established The Deloras Jones Nursing Scholarship Fund in recognition of the commitment and contributions she made to nursing education and excellence in nursing practice in the Kaiser Permanente Health Care Program and to the profession of nursing.

As Kaiser's chief executive nurse leader – a position she held for 15 years – Deloras provided strategic and operational leadership for all of nursing in California, both northern and southern regions. She also served as the corporate nurse, supporting the program leadership. Prior to her regional leadership role, she was the chief nursing officer for the San Francisco hospital and founder of the FAMCP Program – an innovative early hospital discharge option for mother and her new born infant.

After retiring from Kaiser, Deloras founded the California Institute for Nursing & Health Care (CINHC) – now known as HealthImpact. This independent not-for-profit organization serves as the state's nursing workforce center. Deloras retired from this position in November 2012. She has continued engagement in the profession as a consultant on projects that focus on education redesign and increasing access to health care in rural California.

Deloras has once again returned to Kaiser Permanente, serving as a member of Northern California's Regional Life Care Planning Council and as President of the Board of Directors of the Kaiser Foundation School of Nursing Alumni Association. She is also leading the "Continuing the Legacy" endeavor, a partnership between the Alumni Association and KP's northern California Nurse Scholars Academy, where they've published an article, produced award winning videos and now publishing a book about the history and legacy of the Kaiser Foundation School of Nursing.

Deloras received her nursing diploma from the Kaiser Foundation School of Nursing, Baccalaureate in Nursing from Columbia Union College, and Masters in Nursing from the University of California in San Francisco.

Alfonso DNP, RN, PhD(h), NEA-BC, FNAP

Executive Director for Professional Practice, Leadership Development and Research for Kaiser Permanente (KP) and the Founding Executive Director of the KP Scholars Academy in Oakland, California (KP NCAL). In his current role, he leads several nationally recognized programs, including the Exemplary Clinical Practice Partnership Award, granted by the American Association of Colleges of Nursing (AACN) in 2018 and a Telly Award in 2017 for a documentary he produced on KP's 70-Year Legacy of Disruptive Innovation in American Nursing.

Dr. D'Alfonso received his Doctor of Nursing Practice (DNP) with a focus in executive leadership from the University of San Francisco (USF), where he serves as Adjunct Faculty for the School of Nursing and Health Professions. He is a board-certified nurse executive (NEA-BC), WCSI Certified Caritas Coach®, Master HeartMath Executive Trainer (HMET), and a Distinguished Fellow of the Nursing Academies of Practice (FNAP). Jim has published extensively, including his scholarly work on "Aligning theory and evidence-based practice to enhance human flourishing in nurse executives," as well as over 30 articles and book chapters on leadership, nursing theory and clinical best practices. His recent scholarly interests include strategy and workforce development, quantum caring leadership, theory integration into clinical practice, and illuminating synergies between DNP and PhD prepared nurses to advance professional practice, health systems performance and quality patient outcomes.

Jim is president-elect of the Beta Gamma Chapter of Sigma Theta Tau honor society at the University of San Francisco. In 2015, Jim was awarded an Honorary Doctorate in Caring Science by Dr. Jean Watson, honoring his career-long devotion to transformative leadership, scholarly teaching, and practices in human caring. As an early member of Watson's International Caritas Consortia (ICC), he helped champion the articulation of ontological competencies of caring literacy and other innovative approaches to bridge theory and praxis. Jim was appointed founding Chief Nurse Executive and Chief Operating Officer for Watson Caring Science Institute in 2008. During his tenure with WCSI, Jim was responsible for the launch of the Caritas Coach Education Program (CCEP), development of WCSI's prestigious global faculty, and continued expansion of original research and evidence-informed best practices to foster caregiver resilience and health systems transformation.

As an international scholar and keynote speaker, Jim has conducted workshops, consulted, and lectured worldwide for over 30 years, including the Philippines, Japan, Italy, Denmark, Norway, the United Kingdom and Canada.

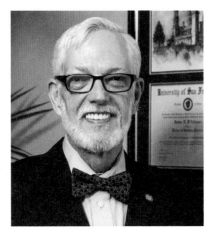

Jim D'Alfonso, DNP, RN, PhD(h), NEA-BC, FNAP

Executive Director, Professional Excellence
The KP Scholars Academy,
Kaiser Foundation Hospitals and Health Plan,
Oakland, California

Adjunct Faculty, University of San Francisco SONHP,
San Francisco, California

Key Locations & Timeline

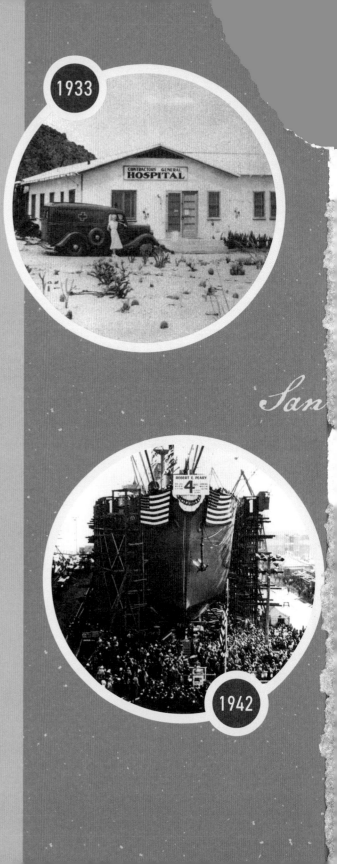

1933
1942
San

1933 Betty Runyen goes to work at Contractors General in Desert Center near Indio.

1938 Sidney Garfield, MD started at Grand Coulee Dam, Washington.

1942 Permanente Foundation established. Kaiser shipyards in Richmond & Washington, operating at full force.

1945 Sidney Garfield, MD, proposed a 3-year school of nursing.

1947 Permanente School of Nursing established in Oakland (Piedmont Hotel). Dorthea Daniels hired to direct school.

1950 Charter class of registered nurses graduate.

1951 The Board of Nursing granted approval for affiliation in tuber-culosis nursing and rehabilitation nursing at Kaiser Foundation Hospital, Vallejo, and the Kabat-Kaiser Institute in Santa Monica. Granted an approval for an eight-week experience in industrial nursing at the Permanente Hospital Fontana.

1953 School of Nursing separates from the Kaiser Foundation Hospital and became an independent organization with its own director and board of trustees. The name of the school changes to Kaiser Foundation School of Nursing (KFSN). The National League for Nursing accredits the school. Marguerite MacLean becomes director of school.

1958 All Santa Monica rehabilitation nursing students are trans-ferred to Kaiser Foundation Hospital in Vallejo. Josephine Coppedge becomes director of school.

1965 A special committee was formed to investigate how Kaiser Foundation School of Nursing could transition from a diploma program to a degree-granting four-year college.

1967 KFSN becomes first diploma school in California to provide an AA degree. Student scores in State Board Examinations ranked top in medical, surgical, and pediatric nursing in the state of California.

1973 Board of Trustees made decision to close the school of nursing.

1976 The school graduated its last and largest class. School closes.